1989

University of St. Francis
G 174.2 F612

W9-AOX-144

3 0301 00055905 0

Ethics Consultation in Health Care

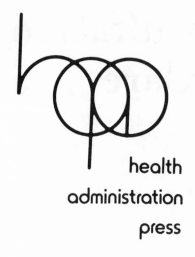

health
administration
press

Editorial Board

John R. Griffith
The University of Michigan

Robert Brook
The Rand Corporation

Douglas A. Conrad
University of Washington

Stephen M. Davidson
Boston University

Judith Feder
Georgetown University

R. Hopkins Holmberg
*Aga Khan Hospital
Nairobi, Kenya*

Rosalie Kane
University of Minnesota

William L. Kissick
The University of Pennsylvania

W. Richard Scott
Stanford University

*Health Administration Press is a
division of the Foundation of the American
College of Healthcare Executives. The
Editorial Board is a cooperative activity
of the Association for Health Services
Research, The University of Michigan,
and the Foundation of the American
College of Healthcare Executives and
selects publications for the Health
Administration Press imprint. The Press
was established in 1972 with the support
of the W.K. Kellogg Foundation.*

Ethics Consultation in Health Care

Edited by
John C. Fletcher
Norman Quist
Albert R. Jonsen

LIBRARY
College of St. Francis
JOLIET, ILLINOIS

Health Administration Press
Ann Arbor, Michigan 1989

Copyright ©1989 by the Foundation of the American College of Healthcare Executives. Printed in the United States of America. All rights reserved. This book or parts thereof may not be reproduced in any form without written permission of the publisher. Opinions and views expressed in this book are those of the author and do not necessarily reflect those of the Foundation of the American College of Healthcare Executives.

Library of Congress Cataloging-in-Publication Data

Ethics consultation in health care / edited by John C.
  Fletcher, Norman Quist, and Albert R. Jonsen.
  p.   cm.
  Includes bibliographies and index.
  ISBN 0-910701-39-3
  1. Medical ethics.   I. Fletcher, John C.   II. Quist,
Norman.   III. Jonsen, Albert R.
  [DNLM: 1. Consultants.   2. Ethics, Medical.
W 50 E842]
R724.E8215   1989
174'.2 − dc20
DNLM/DLC
for Library of Congress   89-11210   CIP

Health Administration Press
A Division of the Foundation of the
  American College of Healthcare Executives
1021 East Huron Street
Ann Arbor, Michigan 48104-9990
(313)764-1380

G
174.2
F612

Contents

134,792

List of Contributors

TERRENCE F. ACKERMAN, PH.D. is Professor and Chairman of the Department of Human Values and Ethics, College of Medicine, University of Tennessee, Memphis. Dr. Ackerman regularly provides ethics case consultations in a variety of clinical services at the medical school. He is also Chairman of the Ethics Advisory Committee, Regional Medical Center at Memphis.

MAXWELL BOVERMAN, M.D. was a consultant to the Bioethics Program of the National Institutes of Health's Clinical Center from 1978 to 1989. He is Clinical Professor of Psychiatry and Internal Medicine at The University of Virginia School of Medicine and serves on the Advisory Committee of its Center for Biomedical Ethics. He is a member of the Board of Directors of the Society for Bioethics Consultation. Dr. Boverman also has a private practice in psychiatry.

ANNE J. DAVIS, PH.D. is Professor at the School of Nursing, University of California, San Francisco. She conducts ethics rounds with hospital staff and acts as ethics consultant to several organizations, including the San Francisco Bay Area Alzheimer's Association.

JAMES F. DRANE, PH.D. is the Russell B. Roth Professor of Clinical Medical Ethics at Edinboro University of Pennsylvania. Recipient of the Distinguished Teaching Chair of Pennsylvania, he has also received numerous grants and fellowships.

In addition to his teaching responsibilities, he provides clinical consultations for Pennsylvania hospitals and nursing homes.

EDMUND G. HOWE, M.D., J.D. is Associate Professor of Psychiatry at the Uniformed Services University of the Health Sciences, F. Edward Hébert School of Medicine. He has directed the school's programs in medical ethics since 1977 and provides consultation primarily to military medical centers in the Washington, DC area.

RUTH B. PURTILO, PH.D. is Henry Knox Sherrill Professor of Medical Ethics and Director of the Program in Ethics at the Massachusetts General Hospital Institute of Health Professions. In addition, she is Ethicist in Residence at Massachusetts General Hospital in Boston. Dr. Purtilo has also served as a hospital ethics consultant at the University of Nebraska Medical Center. She is a founding member of the Society for Bioethics Consultation.

JOHN A. ROBERTSON, J.D. is the Baker & Botts Professor of Law at the University of Texas School of Law at Austin. He has written widely on law and medicine and bioethics issues, including the book *The Rights of the Critically Ill* and numerous articles on reproductive rights. A Fellow of the Hastings Center, he has served on a national Task Force on Organ Transplantation and is a member of the National Institutes of Health Panel on Fetal Tissue Transplantation Research.

LESLIE STEVEN ROTHENBERG, J.D. is Associate Professor of Medicine in the Division of Pulmonary and Critical Care Medicine, Department of Medicine, UCLA School of Medicine, and Director, Program in Medical Ethics, UCLA Medical Center, Los Angeles. A Fellow of the Hastings Center, he has worked as a clinical ethicist for 11 years.

DONNIE J. SELF, PH.D. is Professor in the Department of Humanities in Medicine as well as the Department of Philosophy and the Department of Pediatrics, Texas A&M University.

He has been a frequent contributor to the literature on clinical ethics and was a guest editor of a special issue of *Theoretical Medicine* devoted to clinical ethics.

JOY D. SKEEL, R.N., M.Div. is Associate Professor of Medical Humanities in the Department of Psychiatry, Medical College of Ohio, Toledo. She is the author of articles on medical ethics published in both medical and medical ethics journals. She is a member of the Council of the Society for Health and Human Values.

Introduction

Ethics Consultation in Health Care: Rationale and History

John C. Fletcher, Norman Quist, and Albert R. Jonsen

Ethics consultation is the provision of specialized help in identifying, analyzing, and resolving ethical problems that arise in
clinical care. "Clinical care" refers to all types of health care
given by licensed health professionals, including outpatient,
long-term, and chronic care. Clinical research is an important
part of the clinical setting. In the United States and Canada
today, ethics consultation in health care is a growing service,
usually provided as one feature of an ethics program within an
institution.

There are various ways to provide ethics consultations.
Some institutions or departments designate one individual as
the ethics consultant. Others create an interdisciplinary team for
consultation. Perhaps the most prevalent method is to offer consultation by an ethics committee or by a designated subgroup of
the committee. However, one important feature that all have in
common is that they offer services without charge to those who
request them. We know of no institution that charges fees to
patients for ethics consultation. However, some consultants
have incorporated in the private sector and render services for a
fee to hospitals or health maintenance organizations.

The backgrounds of the contributors to this book illustrate
the diversity of professional backgrounds among ethics consultants. With one exception, the contributors are all actively
involved in giving ethics consultation in health care settings.
They are lawyer-ethicists who are active in clinical situations
(Rothenberg), ethicists who are employed by medical schools

and their teaching hospitals (Ackerman, Skeel, Self, Fletcher, Purtilo, Drane, and Jonsen), a nurse-ethicist (Davis), a physician-lawyer who is also an ethicist (Howe), and a psychiatrist with expertise in consulting with bioethicists (Boverman). John Robertson, a lawyer who is very familiar with issues in bioethics, has contributed a chapter on legal aspects of ethics consultation.

Some chapters were originally papers presented at the First National Conference on Ethics Consultation in Health Care, cosponsored by the Clinical Center of the National Institutes of Health (NIH) and the Division of Medical Ethics of the University of California at San Francisco. This conference met in Bethesda, Maryland on October 7–8, 1985. Following the conference, additional authors were invited to contribute chapters to the book. A preconference questionnaire, completed by 38 (of 53) participants, is included as an appendix at the end of this book, along with a summary of findings.

Costs of the conference were supported by the Warren G. Magnuson Clinical Center and the Office of Protection from Research Risks (NIH), the Eberhard Foundation, and the Blue Cross–Blue Shield Association. A grant from the Kaiser Foundation Health Plan supported the costs of editing and publication of the book.

The remainder of this introduction is divided into three sections. First, we provide actual cases to help the reader appreciate the kinds of problems which ethics consultants are asked to address. These cases may also be useful for new groups of consultants or new ethics committees to explore together for practice. Second, we briefly describe the field of biomedical ethics that undergirds ethics consultation. Finally, we conclude with a brief history of ethics consultation in the United States and Canada to help readers understand the origins and current context of this activity.

CASE EXAMPLES

The cases below illustrate the nature and range of ethical problems which arise in the clinical setting. These cases were referred to the Ethics Consultation Service of the University of Virginia's Medical Center in 1987–88. Some facts have been changed to respect confidentiality.

CASE 1: "I DON'T UNDERSTAND, BUT I DON'T KNOW HOW TO ASK."

The patient, a 40-year-old woman with breast cancer, is to have a partial mastectomy, followed by a course of chemotherapy. Her nurse enters her room and asks her if all of her questions were answered in the almost hour-long meeting with the cancer surgeon. The patient says, "No, there are several things I don't understand, but I don't know how to ask." Some questioning reveals that the patient could not read the consent document that explained the risks and benefits of surgery. How should the nurse respond to this problem of informed consent?

CASE 2: "I DON'T WANT A NEEDLE IN MY BONE."

The patient, a 38-year-old diabetic and alcohol abuser, has been admitted to the hospital many times in a diabetic coma due to complications of noncompliance with treatment and diet. A blood test shows an abnormal number of white cells. Is this due to a suppression of his bone marrow because of alcohol abuse, or is it an early sign of leukemia? His physician needs some of his bone marrow for testing. Bone marrow is obtained by inserting a needle into the hip several times, after a local anesthetic. The patient refuses, saying, "I don't want a needle in my bone." Should the doctor respect the patient's refusal or involve others, including his family, in an attempt to persuade him to comply?

CASE 3: "IS HE COMPETENT TO DECIDE?"

A 17-year-old intoxicated youth is seriously injured around the chest and abdomen in a car accident. He is brought to the emergency room. He has no identification. Physicians need to do a series of radiographic tests, some of which are invasive and involve the swallowing of barium, to assess the extent of his abdominal injuries. He is belligerent and refuses the tests. A physician asks, "Is he competent to decide?" Another points out that delay could have serious consequences, even death. Should they coerce him to agree to the tests?

CASE 4: "SHOULD HER HUSBAND KNOW THE TRUTH?"

The child was born with cystic fibrosis, a hereditary disease which causes cysts and too much fibrous tissue in glandular organs like the pancreas and lungs. Excess mucous secretions cause a blocking of the lungs and pancreatic ducts. The disease is caused by one gene inherited from each parent, which means that both parents of a child with the disease are carriers of the cystic fibrosis gene. The mother confides in the genetic counselor who comes to see her that the biological father of the child is a man other than her husband. Yet her husband now falsely believes that he has a gene for cystic fibrosis. The counselor returns to her office and asks the physicians in the genetics program, "Should her husband know the truth?"

CASE 5: "ABSOLUTELY PROMISE ME THAT YOU WILL NOT TELL ANYONE IF I HAVE AIDS, ESPECIALLY MY MOTHER."

A 30-year-old, single, homosexual man, successful in his profession, is admitted to the hospital with a persistent cough, fever, and swollen lymph glands. His x-rays and blood tests show that he has a form of pneumonia often associated with acquired immune deficiency syndrome (AIDS). His physician asks his consent to test his blood for antibodies to the AIDS virus and explains how the test is done. The man becomes very agitated and asks the doctor to make him a promise. He says, "Absolutely promise me that you will not tell anyone if I have AIDS, especially my mother. Unless you make this promise, I will not permit you to do the test." How should the physician respond to this request for absolute privacy and confidentiality?

CASE 6: "WHY CAN'T WE DONATE ORGANS?"

Ultrasound (a way of visualizing the fetus by sound waves transmitted onto a screen) at seven months of pregnancy reveals that a couple's expected baby has a serious birth defect, anencephaly. The entire forebrain is missing and, if not still-born, the child will die within a few days of birth. However, the brainstem (hindbrain) is intact, and the infant will be able to breathe on its own. Since nothing can be done to treat this devastating birth defect, the customary practice after birth is to allow the baby to die without any intervention other than warmth and comfort. The expectant mother's first thought is to donate the baby's organs to other infants who would die without them. However, an organ donor must be "brain dead" by a definition based on death of the whole brain, including the brainstem. If physicians wait for the infant to die without putting in a breathing tube or other measures, the organs will be damaged by loss of blood and oxygen. Physicians discourage the parents from the hope of donating. They are unwilling to use abortion to end the pregnancy. They ask, "Why can't we donate organs when they are so desperately needed?"

CASE 7: "WHAT ARE WE SUPPOSED TO DO WHEN PHYSICIANS AND FAMILY DISAGREE ABOUT STOPPING LIFE SUPPORTS?"

A 68-year-old widowed patient, resident of a nursing home due to multiple strokes, is brought to the hospital unconscious and with a high fever. He cannot breathe on his own so, in the emergency room, a breathing tube is inserted. He has not spoken or communicated with anyone since his strokes two years ago. He is transferred to the intensive care unit and treated with several antibiotics, but physicians are unable to discover the true source of infection. His two sons and a daughter arrive at the hospital from various parts of the country. They tell the doctors that their father never made his wishes clear about what he wanted done in this kind of situation. They also say that they never talked about this issue with him before his strokes. After a week, the patient has not responded to treatment and becomes steadily worse. His physicians see that further treatment is futile. They recommend to his children that the breathing machine be removed and, if his heart stops, that he be allowed to die without massaging his chest or restarting his heart by electroshock. They need to write a do-not-resuscitate (DNR) order on his medical chart to inform all physicians and nurses of this step. Several attempts to explain the futility of treatment meet with the same response. His sons object to the DNR, saying, "Where there is life, there is hope. This is our belief. We want him coded (resuscitated) until he is brain dead." A physician asks a nurse, "What are we supposed to do when physicians and family disagree about stopping life supports?"

CASE 8: "I WANT TO DIE; MY LIFE IS OVER."

A 35-year-old quadriplegic (paralyzed in the arms and legs) man, injured in an auto accident two years ago, is brought to the hospital by his wife because he refuses to eat or drink. He refuses all medical treatment in the hospital, including food and water by mouth or intravenously. He says to a psychiatrist, "I want to die; my life is over." The psychiatrist, who finds the patient to be rational but significantly depressed, faces the question, "Do I recommend that his refusal be accepted or do I recommend a legal hearing to seek an order to treat in spite of the patient's refusal?"

CASE 9: "SHOULD THE COST OF HEALTH CARE COUNT ETHICALLY?"

A 12-month-old infant, who was born with severe respiratory disease, neurological problems, and possible heart problems, has been a patient in the pediatric intensive care unit for virtually his whole life. The child's mother refuses to allow a cardiac catheterization because she fears that physicians will use the results to recommend that treatment be stopped. However, it is very doubtful that the child will ever leave the hospital. The mother has three other children and very little income. The cost of care is supported by state funds through Medicaid. The cost of intensive care is $1,100 per day. In a review of the case, a medical resident asks, "Should the cost of health care count ethically?"

CASE 10: "CAN WE RATION HEALTH CARE ETHICALLY?"

The administrator of a newly constructed replacement hospital, which is to be opened soon, faces the task of making budget allocations to each major department and clinical service prior to the move to the new hospital. He realizes that the budget allocations will greatly restrict the scope of services provided by some departments and services. He searches for some rationale — based on justice and fairness, yet still compatible with the goals of medicine — to help him make his choices. He asks, "Can we ethically ration health care and not harm patients or services?"

BIOMEDICAL ETHICS

Ethics is the search for practical wisdom, which is sorely needed in approaching cases like those above. The basic questions of ethics, in any field of human conduct, are: What should be done? And why? What reasons support the action? Ethics endeavors to answer these fundamental questions by pursuing two goals: understanding and guidance. Ethics seeks to understand the scope and grounds of our duties and our ideals, and it seeks to guide us to make morally correct decisions: to do what is right and avoid what is wrong. The aim of the field of biomedical ethics is to understand and guide, in a general way, the variety of ethical problems facing health care professionals, patients, and patients' families.

Medical ethics is an ancient field. Biomedical ethics (from *bios*, the Greek word for "life") aims to promote understanding and provide guidance for decision makers regarding ethical issues in the whole spectrum of the life sciences (e.g., molecular biology, human genetics, and clinical research), and their application to human problems. Biomedical ethics, as taught in the clinical setting, must provide understanding and guidance for the most frequent and difficult problems confronting health care workers who care for patients. Biomedical ethics has received increasing attention in our society over the past 25 years owing to rapid and far-reaching technological developments in medical care, some of which figure in the cases above.

Biomedical ethics, as a field, must provide understanding and guidance in approaching these frequent and difficult ethical problems in clinical care: (1) informed consent to treatment, (2) refusal of treatment, (3) determining the patient's capacity to make health care decisions, (4) disclosure or truth-telling dilemmas, (5) privacy and confidentiality, (6) controversial new options in biomedical science, (7) foregoing life-sustaining treatments, (8) medical care of the terminally ill patient, (9) cost-containment methods and the ethical issues raised, and (10) access to health care and allocation of scarce resources. A basic course in biomedical ethics for those engaging in ethics consultation must communicate (a) a basic understanding of the causes and dynamics of such problems, (b) sound ethical guidance in approaching such cases, and (c) the ethical and legal principles which ground the approach to cases. Because the facts of each case will differ, one cannot know in advance of an actual case precisely what is ethically sound and unsound. However, the study of biomedical ethics does provide the grounds from which one approaches each new case. Biomedical ethics begins with the most familiar kind of ethical problems arising in the clinical setting and reaches to those on the creative edges of biomedical research.

ETHICS CONSULTATION: ROOTS AND PRESENT CONTEXT

A historical account of ethics consultation must include these elements: (1) the ancient practice of consultation in medicine, (2) historical parallels in considerations of ethical problems by specialists in religious traditions, (3) the growing ethical complexity in research and medicine after World War II in developed and developing nations, (4) reforms in research ethics, (5) the introduction of medical humanities and bioethics programs in academic medical centers and large teaching hospitals, and (6) encouragement of ethics consultation in significant legal opinions and by national commissions.

Asking for consultation about problems in patient care is a solidly grounded precept in medical ethics. The Hippocratic writings direct physicians in difficulty over a patient and "in the dark through inexperience" to urge "the calling in of others, in order to learn by consultation the truth about the case, and . . . that there may be fellow workers to afford abundant help."[1] The author of this section of the Hippocratic writings also notes (in one translation): "No matter how much help you have you can never have enough." This ancient advice surely applies to ethics consultation!

Thomas Percival's *Medical Ethics*, first published in 1803, urges British physicians to seek help by consultation with others about the problems in long and difficult cases.[2] Percival prescribes approaches to the resolution of conflict between physicians who disagree, when these conflicts threaten the best interests of the patient. The first (1847) and latest (1980) texts of the code of ethics of the American Medical Association also direct physicians to seek consultation.[3,4] Although the codes refer primarily to medical problems for which consultation is needed, the text presumably does not exclude ethics consultation, if such help is available.

Physicians have sought help from one another, or from trusted personal nonmedical advisers, like the clergy, with difficult ethical problems that arise in patient care. Historical precedents for ethics consultation are found in the extensive traditions of rabbinic and moral-theological scholarship on medicine, health, and illness that underlie contemporary interactions between physicians and specialists in Jewish law and Roman Catholic moral theology and canon law.[5,6] These traditions are still very much alive, especially in Jewish and Catholic hospitals and health care systems. However, the emergence of ethics consultants or clinical ethics consultants in contemporary, secular health care institutions is clearly a recent development. How did this development come about and why?

The ethics of medicine and research are multidimensional: they involve more technical options, more choices, no single moral vision to unify the many moral traditions challenged by such choices, and more emphasis on patient autonomy and patient rights. Physicians and their patients are confronted with more ethical complexity today than in the past. The growing ethical complexity in research and practice after World War II is easily documented by (1) the vast literature devoted to such problems in many nations, (2) reports and recommendations of national commissions and working parties mandated by governments to analyze moral conflicts occasioned by science and medicine (e.g., selection of transplant and dialysis recipients, proper use of genetic information, decisions to forego life-sustaining treatment, euthanasia, and new reproductive technologies), and (3) the public and private support given to institutions founded to study such problems, including the Hastings Center and the Kennedy Institute of Ethics in the United States, and comparable institutions in Canada, such as the Center for Bioethics (Montreal) and the Westminster Institute for Ethics and Human Values (London).[7]

Against a background of growing ethical complexity in medicine and research, three historical experiences directly influenced the origins of ethics consultation in health care: (1) prior group consideration of research, (2) the influence of the medical humanities and bioethics movements in the United States and Canada, and (3) significant legal opinions that influenced the formation of hospital ethics committees.

ORIGINS IN REFORMS IN RESEARCH ETHICS

There are at least three positive outcomes that ground and validate ethics consultation: first, a higher degree of impartiality in assessing ethical problems and options; second, the increase in knowledge of ethics, self, and others that often accompanies a well-conducted consultation; and third, the benefits that result from a consultation that combines respect-for the patient's and family's interests with optimal participation by key decision makers.

These benefits of clinical consultation were considered in earlier reforms in clinical research ethics, especially the quest for impartiality that found expression in the practice of prior group review of research. The reforms of the 1960s and early 1970s achieved a higher degree of protection for research subjects and researchers, who are also at risk to be exploited due to societal and group pressures for health benefits and achievement. Would anyone seriously want to return to a period when *only* researchers could decide on the premier ethical questions in research, such as: Should this project be done at all? What are its risks and benefits? The ethical megadisasters that resulted from judgments made by self-interested researchers were too harmful and numerous to go uncorrected by continuing a tradition of only scientific peer review.[8-10] Physicians in the previous generation (1950–70) were trained in academic centers that adopted changes in research practices by 1966 and beyond. Contemporary physicians (1970–90) were trained in academic centers where prior group review of the ethics of research projects is an established practice required by federal and state statutes. The highest ethical good resulting from these regulations is a higher degree of impartiality in the most important moral judgments about research. This is so widely recognized today that any proposal for human subjects research in the United States and Canada, regardless of its institutional setting, would be judged ethically defective without such consideration. Well-conducted meetings of review groups are also likely to increase knowledge of ethics, self, and others, as well as to increase respect for the prospective subject's rights and freedom to choose to be in research at all. The point is that without a background of these changes in medical *research* ethics, physicians would not be as open as they are to asking for help with ethical problems in medical *practice*. The difference is that researchers *must* ask for help in assessing the ethical adequacy of a project; in the clinical setting, physicians *may* ask for ethics consultation.

ORIGINS IN MEDICAL HUMANITIES AND BIOETHICS PROGRAMS

The first ethics consultants in the 1960s and 1970s were founders of programs of medical humanities or medical ethics in teaching hospitals. In addition to their teaching, they were requested to help with ethical problems in cases involving patients.[11,12] The humanities programs were innovations in medical education for a stronger emphasis on the study of the humanities and ethics.[13,14] As these teaching programs became more integrated in academic medical institutions, it was only a matter of time before ethics consultations became one of the major vehicles for teaching medical ethics to house staff and students. What better way to teach than from the living example?[15,16]

ORIGINS IN LEGAL OPINIONS

The origins of ethics committees have been thoroughly documented in legal opinions and proposed federal rules that encouraged such groups to become involved in decisions to forego life-sustaining treatment in adults like Karen Ann Quinlan (1976) and infants like Infant Doe of Bloomington, Indiana (1982) and Infant Doe of New York (1983).[17,18] These and other cases created a significant body of legal opinions and principles in choices to forego life-sustaining treatment.[19] Most of the written opinions of the majority have stressed the need for hospitals to provide means to resolve similar problems close to the bedside with the persons most directly involved. Reflecting on the use of the courts to resolve such problems, the President's Commission for the Study of Ethical Problems in Medicine and Biomedical and Behavioral Research recommended in 1983 that courts should be used as decision makers for incompetent individuals requiring medical treatment only as a last resort.[20] The commission recommended that health care institutions were responsible

> to ensure that there are appropriate procedures to enhance patients' competence, to provide for the designation of surrogates, to guarantee that patients are adequately informed, to overcome the influence

of dominant institutional biases, to provide review of decision making, and to refer cases to the courts appropriately. (p. 4)

The commission intended that the consultation function in hospitals be especially protective of the interests of patients who lack decision-making capacity, especially in the review of life and death decisions made by their surrogates and physicians. The commission added that

the medical staff, along with the trustees and administrators of health care institutions, should explore and evaluate various formal and informal administrative arrangements for review and consultation, such as "ethics committees," particularly for decisions that have life-or-death consequences. (p. 5)

When ethics committees appeared, it was expected that these bodies should develop the capacity for consultation. The state of Maryland passed a law in 1987 requiring that each licensed hospital have a "patient care advisory committee" to give guidance on request in cases involving choices to forego life-sustaining treatment.[21] Maryland is the only state to require such committees in each hospital.

PRESENT CONTEXT: ETHICS PROGRAMS IN HOSPITALS

Ethics consultation has roots in earlier reforms in research ethics, medical education, and conflicts about patient care ethics that reached the courts and legislatures. Today, ethics consultation is one of several aspects of ethics programs in many contemporary hospitals in the United States and Canada. We use the term "program" to emphasize the institutional setting of ethics consultation, necessary related activities, and the institution's responsibility (as stated by the President's Commission) to support and provide for such activities. The program, especially in academic medical centers, can also continue to take the form of medical humanities, which includes attention to ethics. The four features of an ethics program are (1) a hospital ethics committee as the focus and forum for ethical concerns in the hospital, (2) a capacity to give ethics consultation for cases, on request, either prospectively or retrospectively, (3) an educational program in biomedical ethics that serves the hospital staff, students, and the community, and (4) access to one or more individuals with advanced education in biomedical ethics who serve as resource persons in the other three aspects of the program. Ethics consultation in a health care institution must not be separated from the need to balance and work simultaneously in these four program areas.

We feel fortunate to share in the formation of a new field and to have this opportunity to present it to the reader.

REFERENCES

1. Selections from the Hippocratic Corpus. In *Ethics in Medicine*, edited by Stanley J. Reiser, Arthur J. Dyck, and William J. Curran. Cambridge, MA: MIT Press, 1977.
2. Percival, Thomas. *Medical Ethics*, 3rd edition. Oxford: John Henry Parker, 1849.
3. American Medical Association. "First Code of Medical Ethics. Proceedings of the National Medical Convention, 1846–1847." In *Ethics in Medicine*, edited by Stanley J. Reiser, Arthur J. Dyck, and William J. Curran, 26–34. Cambridge, MA: MIT Press, 1977.
4. American Medical Association. *Current Opinions of the Judicial Council*. Chicago: American Medical Association, 1981.
5. Trainin, Isaac N., and Rosner, Fred. "Jewish Codes and Guidelines." In *Encyclopedia of Bioethics*, edited by Warren T. Reich, 1428–30. New York: Free Press, 1978.
6. Curran, Charles E. "Roman Catholicism." In *Encyclopedia of Bioethics*, edited by Warren T. Reich, 1522–34. New York: Free Press, 1978.
7. Williams, John R. *Biomedical Ethics in Canada*. Lewiston, NY: The Edwin Mellen Press, n.d. ISBN 0-88946-149-X.
8. Beecher, Henry K. "Ethics in Clinical Research." *New England Journal of Medicine* 274 (1966): 1354–60.
9. Pappworth, M. H. *Human Guinea Pigs*. London: Routledge and Kegan Paul, 1967.
10. Fletcher, John C. "The Evolution of the Ethics of Informed Consent." In *Research Ethics*, edited by Kåre Berg and Knut E. Tranöy, 187–228. New York: Alan R. Liss, 1985.
11. Jonsen, Albert R. "Can an Ethicist Be a Consultant?" In *Frontiers in Medical Ethics*, edited by Virginia Abernethy, 157–71. Cambridge, MA: Ballinger, 1980.

12. Levine, Melvin D.; Scott, Lee; and Curran, William J. "Ethics Rounds in a Children's Medical Center: Evaluation of a Hospital-Based Program for Continuing Education in Medical Ethics." *Pediatrics* 60 (1977): 202-8.

13. Pellegrino, Edmund D. "Human Values and the Medical Curriculum." *Journal of the American Medical Association* 209 (1969): 1349-53.

14. Pellegrino, Edmund D. "Reform and Innovation in Medical Education: The Role of Ethics." In *The Teaching of Medical Ethics*, edited by Robert M. Veatch, Willard Gaylin, and Councilman Morgan, 150-65. Hastings-on-Hudson, NY: The Hastings Center, 1973.

15. Pellegrino, Edmund D. "Ethics and the Moment of Clinical Truth." *Journal of the American Medical Association* 239 (1978): 960-61.

16. Siegler, Mark. "A Legacy of Osler: Teaching Ethics at the Bedside." *Journal of the American Medical Association* 239 (1978): 951-56.

17. Cranford, Ronald E., and Doudera, A. Edward. "The Emergence of Institutional Ethics Committees." In *Institutional Ethics Committees and Health Care Decision Making*, edited by Ronald E. Cranford and A. Edward Doudera, 5-21. Ann Arbor, MI: Health Administration Press, 1984.

18. Hosford, Bowen I. *Bioethics Committees*. Rockville, MD: Aspen Publications, 1986.

19. Areen, Judith; King, Patricia A.; Goldberg, Steven; and Capron, Alexander M. *Law, Medicine, and Science*. Mineola, NY: The Foundation Press, 1984.

20. President's Commission for the Study of Ethical Problems in Medicine and Biomedical and Behavioral Research. *Decisions to Forego Life Sustaining Treatment*. Washington, DC: U.S. Government Printing Office, 1983.

21. Maryland law.

Part I

The Role of the Ethics Consultant

INTRODUCTION

Part I explores the role of the ethics consultant. How should this role be defined? Upon which concept of ethics should the role be based? How do ethics consultants in the field understand their role? The three chapters in Part I deal directly with these questions.

Leslie Steven Rothenberg (in one of the previously mentioned papers prepared for a 1985 NIH-sponsored conference on ethics consultation) argues that the role of the consultant in ethics must be "clinical" (i.e., focus on patients and their care by physicians). To merit the term "ethics consultant," Rothenberg suggests, a person must be "involved in the clinical activities of the health care facility in which he or she works." He supports his argument with the results of a historical study of the term "clinical," discusses how the term should be applied in ethics consultation, and explores reactions, including a backlash by some physicians against the use of ethicists in the clinical setting. He also describes how he became a clinical ethicist and the scope of his duties.

Written from the perspective of a philosopher, Terrence F. Ackerman's chapter shows that questions about the role of consultants are inseparable from ideas in basic moral theory or from choices about which social problems the consultant is expected to help ameliorate. He defines the unique function of the ethics consultant as a facilitator of moral inquiry. Then he explores some specific conflicts (analysis vs. answers, reflection vs. action, advocacy vs. impartiality, and critique vs. interpretation) in the consultant's role. Drawing upon his view of the properties of moral inquiry, Ackerman reviews six features of ethics consultation. He concludes that the consultant does not have all the answers, is not a monitor of the clinical care received by the patient, but may legitimately be a "whistle blower." In addition, the consultant must impartially represent the moral interests of all relevant parties, and must have maximum freedom to critically assess existing social rules related to the care of patients.

Joy D. Skeel and Donnie J. Self briefly discuss the history of the rise in interest in clinical ethics. After discussion with colleagues in the field, they organized a project to study how ethicists actually function in the clinical setting. They describe four common views of the ethicist: (1) the consultant called in to make recommendations on patient care in difficult cases, (2) an educator working with providers and students but not with patients, (3) a counselor to providers but not to patients, and (4) a patient advocate who protects patients and defends their rights. They report on the preliminary findings of their study.

1

Clinical Ethicists and Hospital Ethics Consultants: The Nature of the "Clinical" Role

Leslie Steven Rothenberg

> So it is almost necessary, in all controversies and disputations, to imitate the wisdom of the mathematicians, in setting down in the very beginning the definitions of our words and terms, that others may know how we accept and understand them, and whether they concur with us or no. For it cometh to pass, for want of this, that we are sure to end there where we ought to have begun, which is, in questions and differences about words.
>
> —Francis Bacon, *Advancement of Knowledge, 1605*

Clinical ethicist. Medical ethicist. Ethics consultant. Applied bioethicist. These are purportedly labels that describe professional roles and activities, and they often pop up in discussions that contain the adjective *clinical*, as in "clinical setting," "clinical judgment," "clinical medicine," or "clinical role." The noun form of the same word, *clinician*, is usually used to describe physicians.

Writers have used the adjective heavily and the noun more sparingly, but with little effort in either case to define the resulting phrases. They clearly assume that the adjective *clinical* is understood by all who see it as meaning exactly what the writer intended, even though different writers use the word in ways that may have opposite meanings. The reader cannot be certain if clinical connotes a physical or geographical setting (a clinic and a hospital or a physician's office), a type of relationship to patients in such a setting, a relationship to people who

take care of such patients, the problems of patients that caregivers attempt to diagnose and treat, a status or privilege or
institutional categorization given to those who work in a health
care setting, a more general preoccupation with things practical rather than purely theoretical, or some other meaning. In
some contexts, the connection to patients is clear; in others, it
is far less obvious or not present at all.

A failure to define terms may lead to confusion on the
part of those who come into contact with "clinical ethicists" or
"ethics consultants." It may also confuse the holder of such a
title as to the proper nature of his or her role in the institutional
setting. As a contribution to overcoming this semantic muddle,
this chapter will explore the meanings and uses of the adjective
clinical to address the potential roles (and the implications of
those roles) for medical ethicists who teach and consult in a
defined clinical setting. It will also suggest a minimum standard or requirement for any person wishing to call himself or
herself a clinical ethicist or ethics consultant.

I.

An etymological excursion into the history of the word *clinical*
discloses its derivation from Greek, Latin, and French words.
The Greek verb *klinein* (to slope) yielded the derivative noun
kline (a couch or bed) and the adjective *klinikos* (of or belonging
to a bed). The Latin *clinicus* and the French *clinique* refer to a
person who is bedridden and came to mean a physician who
visits patients at their beds.[1,2] An alternative definition of the
modern English adjective refers to one who is "concerned with
observation and treatment of patients rather than medical
theory."[3]

Thus, the original focus of the term *clinical* is the human
patient or, to be historically accurate, the patient's bed. Yet the
adjective can be used in ways that do not directly refer to such
patients, in or out of bed. For example, the Joint Commission
on Accreditation of Hospitals (now the Joint Commission on
Accreditation of Healthcare Organizations) defined the phrase
"clinical privileges" as "permission to render medical care in the

granting institution within well-defined limits, based on the individual's professional license and his experience, competency, ability and judgment."[4] It can be argued, of course, that medical care is rendered to patients, but a veterinarian in a research hospital may be given clinical privileges, thus expanding our customary concept of the word *patient*.

Another illustration of the potential for the word *clinical* to be used in more general and less patient-directed ways is Cassell's discussion of the phrase "clinical meaning," which, he writes, "implies that something can be measured in a practical manner, has predictive and explanatory value, and can thus enter into decision making."[5] Although occurring in a paper that is clearly addressed to medical decision making involving patients, Cassell's definition could be used to discuss the phrase "practical meaning" or some equally general and nonmedical concept. Indeed, another alternative dictionary definition of the word *clinical* is "dispassionately critical,"[6] as in this sentence: "Her published review of the novel was viewed by many readers as devastatingly clinical."

The more typical use of the term, however, clearly focuses on the patient. One well-known internal medicine text defines "clinical information" as encompassing "information obtained by conversing with the patient and his relatives (the history), information obtained by observing and examining the patient (the physical examination), as well as information obtained through laboratory examinations of the patient or specimens obtained from the patient (laboratory tests), and from special procedures such as endoscopy."[7] Similarly, Carlton, a medical sociologist, has defined clinical judgment as "the capacity to make medical decisions based on clinical data (history, physical examination, diagnosis, prognosis), with support from secondary resources, such as the medical literature." Seeking to define what she labels the "clinical reality," Carlton writes that "the clinical perspective entails the evaluation of patient history and physical examination, laboratory data, and available consultants' reports; together they create 'the clinical picture.' It is supported by access to medical literature and the accumulation of clinical experience. The use of the clinical perspective results in the development of 'clinical judgment.' "[8]

Using *clinical* in a patient-related context is consistent with the Hippocratic view that medicine (or as Hippocrates called it, "the art") involves three factors: the patient's history, diagnosis, and prognosis. As Jonsen observes, the role of the physician is then to follow (or, translating from the Greek, "to pull his oar along with") the logical insights gained from such patient-centered information.[9]

Various writers have noted the centrality of the patient in defining the term *clinical ethics*. Jonsen, Siegler, and Winslade have defined clinical ethics as "the identification, analysis, and resolution of moral problems that arise in the care of a particular patient."[10] Siegler, in fact, distinguishes what he calls "biomedical ethics" ("greatly concerned with public policy issues") from "clinical ethics" by stating that the latter "focuses on issues that confront the physician in his daily interactions with patients."[11] Kollemorten and colleagues have made the same point in another manner by defining the word *ethical* in the clinical context: "A clinical decision has an ethical component, when the doctor bases his/her action (diagnostic, examination or treatment) or his/her information to the patients or others on a value judgment."[12]

The source of clinical information, the "laboratory" of clinical care, is the interaction with the patient. It is essential to the meaning of the word *clinical* as used in a health care setting. As one writer observed, "the most basic unit of the clinical art must happen in the process of a single doctor-patient meeting."[13] Some have sought to distinguish the scientific from the nonscientific (pejoratively, the "hard" from the "soft") dimensions of the clinical interaction with patients. Bosk observes that clinical expertise is "artful," "almost mystical," "a charismatic possession, a gift of grace," "a mystery," whereas scientific evidence is "rational," "technical," "most routine," "known to all."[14] Carlton notes that what she describes as the clinical and legal perspectives of the clinical setting tend to be characterized by "principles of objectification, concreteness, and case-by-case review," while what she calls the "moral perspective" is

characterized by "subjectivity and diffuseness."[15] In such a setting, it is more often lay people, she asserts, who see moral
questions in clinical situations, while physicians often see only
"clinical problems." (If that is an accurate observation, Veatch
might be prepared to argue that what we need are not clinical
ethicists but rather "lay medical ethicists" who can discuss the
choices and values of lay people.[16])

The typical clinical discussion, according to Carlton, is
not based on deontological and teleological considerations,
"even though these may be teased out of clinical practice."[17]
This then raises the issue of whether ethical issues form an
external, unrelated element of clinical practice, or whether (as
Jonsen, Siegler, and Winslade assert) "good clinical medicine is
ethical medicine" and "consists in technical skill together with
its sensitive application to the personal needs of the person
asking for help in the care of his/her health."[18] If, as Pellegrino
suggests, the requirement of a humane physician is to be as
clinically competent as possible,[19] how do ethicists provide
training for physicians and other health care professionals
(and, if desired, the patient-specific consultations on ethical
issues in clinical medicine)? Who is qualified to provide such
training and consultations, and who does the qualifying?

II.

Before one can focus on the qualifications of the teacher and
the methods for teaching, there must be agreement on exactly
what is to be offered. As with the use of the word *clinical*, there
are differing notions of what we mean by our use of the word
ethics in the context of the physician-patient or caregiver-
patient relationship.

There are numerous models of the physician-patient relationship, including the engineering, priestly, collegial, contrac-
tual, and covenantal models originally described by Veatch.[20-22]
Added to these are the models or explanations of clinical decision making offered largely by physicians not involved in the
teaching of ethics.[23]

Models of clinical-ethical decision making have also been

offered. Jonsen and colleagues,[24] Siegler,[25] and Cassell[26] have all endorsed a model involving four general categories by which most considerations arising in a clinical case can be understood and resolved: (1) the indications for medical intervention, (2) patient preferences, (3) "quality of life" factors, and (4) factors external to the immediate physician-patient encounter (including family wishes, economic issues, societal interests, and others). Thomasma has described medical ethics as a symbiotic discipline embracing both medicine and ethics, requiring a six-step process of moral reasoning that enables "right" decisions to be made when they are based on a coherent understanding of both medicine and the values that enter into medical decisions.[27] Pellegrino has argued that both physicians and hospitals need to act as moral agents in their interactions with patients.[28]

Endless pages have been devoted to debating questions such as whether physicians are moral enough to deal with ethical issues in medicine without the help of scientifically impoverished outsiders who do not understand the context for the decision making, whether only philosophers have the training in ethics to be able to teach and consult on these issues, and whether medical ethics is simply applied general ethics.

Historical evidence suggests that there has been a backlash against bioethics and medical ethics by some physicians who saw the involvement of people waving the banner of ethics as intrusive and potentially harmful to the physician-patient relationship. In 1978, one physician wrote frantically that ethicists were the "newest danger on the physician's horizon."[29] Callahan,[30] Caplan,[31] and Clouser[32] have described this backlash thoughtfully, and they have all noted the ethicist's need for clinical/scientific competence when seeking to work in a medical setting. The reactions against the involvement of ethicists continue today. Swales, a British academic physician, argues that because ethical judgments cannot be separated from clinical judgments, and because things clinical are scientific (whereas things ethical are metaphysical), he "cannot accept that there is a discipline of medical ethics which can somehow throw light on what we should do."[33]

Even the seemingly defensive tone of responses by hospital-based philosophers, praising the contribution of ethical theory to medicine, have acknowledged the need for more clinical experience on the part of medical ethics. Arras and Murray, responding to Swales, argued for clinically based medical ethics in which sophistication in dealing with ethical theory is combined with "an appreciation of the empirical details of clinical practice" and "a knowledge of medical facts and medical practice."[34] Ruddick and Finn have also acknowledged the need for such background: "We readily admit the importance of first-hand clinical experience and the risks of semi-ignorant intrusiveness, even if well-intentioned."[35]

A veritable tidal wave of support, not only for ethicists' need for clinical background but also for physicians' need for an ethical background, has been building for over a decade. In 1976, Veatch and Sollitto, writing on medical ethics teaching at that time, commented on the need to involve both patients and physicians in the teaching of medical ethics and the critical need to combine both clinical and ethical skills (possibly by creating a physician-ethicist team to do the teaching).[36] Ingelfinger, himself skeptical about the role of medical ethicists, nevertheless urged in 1975 that ethicists "should spend months at a university hospital," because of the need for greater understanding of physicians by ethicists and vice versa.[37] Churchill commented in 1977 on the benefits ethicists could gain from a better understanding of the clinical context, of the routines of clinical medicine, and of the "tacit level of professional and value components."[38]

In 1978, Jonsen wrote that "ethics in medicine cannot be done well at a distance" and that there is a critical distinction between the ethics *of* medicine ("an attempt to express some symbols which represent an ideal form of medicine's relationship to society and persons") and ethics *in* medicine ("a symbolic expression of that ideal under the constraints of actual social conditions and in conditions of uncertainty of knowledge and indefiniteness of responsibility").[39] Also in 1978, Siegler wrote his classic article on teaching clinical ethics at the bedside. He wrote of the possible division of responsibility between

134,792

LIBRARY
College of St. Francis
JOLIET, ILLINOIS

ethicist-philosophers and physicians in the preclinical and clinical years of undergraduate medical school education. Furthermore, he offered four advantages of teaching at the bedside: "(1) actual cases to maximize personal accountability; (2) reinforcing the relationship between technical competence and ethical decisions; (3) involving the entire health care team; and (4) possibly decreasing the resistance of the medical profession to formal medical ethics."[40]

In 1980, Thomasma published an article describing the program he had established at the University of Tennessee to provide theoretical and clinical training for ethicists, and articulating a rationale for a clinically centered, patient-focused program. "Clinical exposure is necessary at the very least for an understanding of clinical judgment, the pressure to decide and its impact on medical and patient values, the art of the experienced clinician and the role of experiment in modern clinical practice. . . . Medical ethics becomes remote, more like pure ethics, insofar as it becomes removed from helpful, clinical concerns."[41]

That same year, Jonsen wrote of the ethicist as a consultant, one who is "doing ethics" in a way that is "directly relevant to clinical decisions," the ethics consultant as the modern "casuist" who applies principles to cases.[42]

Cassell has written of the benefits of ethical principles demonstrated in a clinical context and the growing interest of physicians in the clinical application of such principles.[43] An article has even appeared in a hospital trade association journal, urging hospital administrators to consider hiring as hospital ethicists only those persons who have some clinical background, because the ethicist should function as an "inside aide, not an outside expert."[44]

Articles by physicians have urged the expansion of clinical education that includes ethics training. Hiatt wrote of the need for such training to help physicians understand their professional responsibility.[45] Clinical ethics has the potential to contribute to the areas of forensic psychiatry[46-48] and geriatric medicine,[49] to mention only two specialty areas.

Ethicists' descriptions of programs for teaching clinical

ethics include: (1) Veatch's description of the Hastings Center–Columbia College of Physicians and Surgeons collaboration,[50] (2) Ruddick's review of the creation of the Society for Philosophy and Public Affairs in New York City in 1969, and their work at Bellevue and Montefiore Hospitals,[51] (3) Siegler and colleagues' assessment of a case studies approach for junior medical students,[52] and (4) Thomasma's previously mentioned description of the University of Tennessee program.[53]

Possible roles or approaches for such clinical ethicists, in both teaching and consulting, have also been analyzed. Veatch was most optimistic in 1973 that certain cases in the Columbia program were being discussed within the clinical conference format then used by medical services on the wards.[54] Pellegrino wrote in 1978 of the possible methods of a clinical ethicist as including "ethical grand rounds, bedside rounds, ethics committees, [and] problem-oriented seminars."[55] Fleischman suggested three promising areas of work: house staff and attending physician education, case consultations, and advice regarding institutional policies.[56]

Such activities are not without their potential hazards, of course. Clouser has warned that the clinical setting may be a difficult place to teach ethics because of the sense of urgency and the lack of time for reflection. He prefers "attending rounds" to "work rounds" for the additional reflective time available and asks whether it is appropriate for the ethicist to see patients with the physician(s).[57] Ruddick suggested that hospital-based philosophers might become absorbed "into the medical center ethos and become collaborators in a flawed system," but that had not been his experience.[58] Pellegrino has cautioned about the need to avoid being intimidated by the complexity and urgency of bedside decisions.[59]

Siegler has advised humanists working in the clinical setting to: "(1) come to clinical medicine with a strong base in your own discipline; (2) learn all you can about medicine; (3) avoid presumptuousness; (4) don't be a reformer; and (5) attend carefully to the ethical issues raised by the presence of a humanist in the clinical setting."[60]

The appropriate educational background and training for

the clinical ethicist position has not been officially pronounced by any organization. Fletcher has noted the possible choices of an ethicist or philosopher, a social scientist, a psychiatrist, a lawyer, or a physician-clinician, offering the suggestion that, regardless of background, the individual must have demonstrated competence in at least one level of Henry Aiken's well-known levels of moral discourse.[61] Siegler clearly prefers the physician-ethicist model[62] and has developed a program at the University of Chicago to provide training for such individuals. Philosophers and theologians may have had the most in-depth training in ethics generally, but as Dyck has noted, medical ethics is a subspecies of ethics, "with a distinctive body of thought and practice . . . not limited to physicians either in general articulation or clinical application."[63] It follows that neither philosophers, theologians, nor physicians should have an exclusive hold on the field of clinical ethics or ethics consultations, although each area of training may offer valuable skills and insight. The issue of whether or not a certification program for clinical ethicists or ethics consultants is desirable and, if so, who should comprise the body of certifiers, will have to be addressed in the future.

It appears that calling a person a clinical ethicist or an ethics consultant requires, at a minimum, that the person be involved in the clinical activities of the health care facility in which he or she works. To be worthy of the title, a clinical ethicist must interact with patients and their families as well as with the caregivers responsible for the patients. The lack of such contact raises significant questions about the ethicist/consultant's understanding of patients' values and concerns (as well as of those of their families or significant others), and about his or her ability to assist the health care team in dealing with issues related to patients' values.

Perhaps it can be argued that an ethicist who is teaching the ethics *of* medicine as opposed to ethics *in* medicine (to use Jonsen's apt phrases) need not see patients to be considered an ethics consultant. This position may distort the traditional notion of a consultant in the clinical setting as a patient-related concept; a better title for such an individual might be *medical* ethicist, without any reference to clinical competence. However, a willingness to rely totally on secondhand information about the patient, when offering advice or raising issues in a consultative situation, would raise serious doubts about the credibility or value of the enterprise. It is important to recognize the significance of titles as well as the value of clinical experience. It is obvious that a medical ethicist might provide helpful advice to a physician or nurse without seeing the patient under discussion, just as a physician in a distant city might provide advice by phone in a difficult case. However, it is his or her clinical experience and competence that justifies the telephone call, and such competence would also prompt the call to the ethicist.

III.

Trained originally as a lawyer, I became interested in medical ethics when I was teaching on a law faculty. My curiosity about a court petition seeking to enforce Karen Quinlan's alleged legal rights as a Roman Catholic to have her ventilator support discontinued gradually led to a fascination with the problems of neurological prognosis and the dilemmas of clinical decision making in hospital intensive care units.

In 1978, a neonatologist invited me to "round" with a neonatal intensive care unit (NICU) team in a very large, academically affiliated community hospital. What began as an educational experience resulted in an invitation to speak to physicians, nurses, and social workers about ethical issues which were emerging in the clinical setting. Separate chance meetings with a neonatologist and a pulmonary specialist at the UCLA Medical Center led to similar opportunities to lead "ethics rounds" in their NICU and respiratory intensive care unit. I continued these activities at both institutions for several years in an informal and volunteer capacity.

In the fall of 1980, I was appointed to the faculty of the Department of Medicine at UCLA in its Division of Pulmonary Diseases. My division chief pressed for the appointment to validate what he felt was the importance of teaching and consulting on ethical issues in the training of physicians at UCLA. I have focused my efforts in teaching clinical ethics primarily on postgraduate physicians (interns, residents, and fellows) and, using Jonsen's phrase, "doing ethics" as a consultant to all of the medical and nursing services at the medical center on a 24-hour on-call basis.

I review and write progress notes in patients' medical records ("charts") and am legally responsible for those entries. At their physicians' requests, I regularly see patients and their families or friends, working directly with them and the health care teams to resolve ethical or value concerns. In addition to speaking at departmental grand rounds and conferences, I conduct weekly "ethics rounds" on critical care and geriatric medicine services. At these rounds, house staff select patients for presentation in light of the specific ethical issues perceived by the medical teams. Nursing team members and social workers assigned to the services attend these rounds, as do the attending physicians for both services. The critical care rounds are also attended by consultation-liaison psychiatry residents who address any psychiatric issues raised in the discussion.

As a member of the heart transplant team and the pediatric bone marrow transplant team, I raise and discuss ethical issues as they arise in the selection and treatment of candidates for these procedures. I am coeditor (with Judith Wilson Ross) of a monthly newsletter on ethical issues in medicine for the faculty, house staff, and medical students at UCLA and a bimonthly newsletter on ethical issues in nursing for the members of the nursing service at the medical center and the students and faculty of the UCLA School of Nursing. The newsletters review recently published articles on medical ethics, emphasizing those that address ethical issues in the clinical setting. In addition, I have encouraged the creation of several ethics committees at the medical center. All of these activities are part of my role as director of the UCLA Medical Center's newly created program in medical ethics, which is designed to reach all health care providers working there and which includes in-service teaching for nurses, social workers, and other health professionals.

The primary focus of all of my work is clinical ethics in the hospital setting, involving both inpatients and outpatients, from neonates to centenarians. Physicians and nurses have become accustomed to seeing me at the bedsides of patients on nights and weekends, which seems to lend some credibility to and greater acceptance of my role. My teaching and consulting are largely done at the bedside, both because I need to study the clinical information and to see the patient to better inform my comments, and because I prefer working in that setting (as opposed to a more distant one). I always inform patients and families of my role and seek their consent for my involvement. I also observe the privacy and confidentiality requirements expected of health care professionals, and I respect the authority of the attending physicians in case consultations.

A person can become involved in the clinical setting and become, for better or worse, a nonphysician clinician. The clinician or clinical ethicist label is both a responsibility and a reminder to be conscious of the realities of the clinical setting and of the humility with which one must discuss complex and problematic value choices in the context of medical decision making.

REFERENCES

1. Partridge, Eric, ed. *Origins: A Short Etymological Dictionary of Modern English*, 2nd ed. London: Routledge and Kegan Paul, 1959.
2. Skeat, Walter W., ed. *An Etymological Dictionary of the English Language*. Oxford: Clarendon Books, 1910.
3. Stein, Jess, ed. *The Random House Dictionary*. New York: Ballantine Books, 1978.
4. Joint Commission on Accreditation of Hospitals. *Accreditation Manual for Hospitals, 1984*. Chicago: Joint Commission on Accreditation of Hospitals, 1983.
5. Cassell, Eric J. "Moral Thought in Clinical Practice." In *Science, Ethics and Medicine*, edited by H. Tristram Engelhardt, Jr. and Daniel Callahan, 147–60. Hastings-on-Hudson, NY: The Hastings Center, 1976.
6. Stein, *The Random House Dictionary*.

7. Harvey, A. McGehee; Johns, Richard J.; McKusick, Victor A.; Owens, Albert H., et al., eds. *The Principles and Practice of Medicine*, 20th ed. New York: Appleton-Century-Crofts, 1980.

8. Carlton, Wendy. *In Our Professional Opinion: The Primacy of Clinical Judgment over Moral Choice*. Notre Dame, IN: University of Notre Dame Press, 1978.

9. Jonsen, Albert R. "Do No Harm: Axiom of Medical Ethics." In *Philosophical Medical Ethics: Its Nature and Significance*, edited by Stuart F. Spicker and H. Tristram Engelhardt, Jr., 27–41. Boston: D. Reidel, 1977.

10. Jonsen, Albert R.; Siegler, Mark; and Winslade, William. *Clinical Ethics*. New York: Macmillan, 1982.

11. Siegler, Mark. "Clinical Ethics and Clinical Medicine." *Archives of Internal Medicine* 139 (1979): 914–15.

12. Kollemorten, I.; Strandberg, C.; Thomsen, B. M.; Wiberg, O., et al. "Ethical Aspects of Clinical Decision-Making." *Journal of Medical Ethics* 7 (1981): 67–69.

13. Coulehan, John L. "Dissecting the Clinical Art." *Pharos* 47 (1984): 21–25.

14. Bosk, Charles L. *Forgive and Remember: Managing Medical Failure*. Chicago: University of Chicago Press, 1979.

15. Carlton, *In Our Professional Opinion*.

16. Veatch, Robert M. "Lay Medical Ethics." *Journal of Medicine and Philosophy* 10 (1985): 1–5.

17. Carlton, *In Our Professional Opinion*.

18. Jonsen, Siegler, and Winslade, *Clinical Ethics*.

19. Pellegrino, Edmund D. "Reform and Innovation in Medical Education: The Role of Ethics." In *The Teaching of Medical Ethics*, edited by Robert M. Veatch, Willard Gaylin, and Councilman Morgan, 150–65. Hastings-on-Hudson, NY: The Hastings Center, 1973.

20. Clouser, K. Danner. "Veatch, May, and Models: A Critical Review and a New View." In *The Clinical Encounter*, edited by Earl E. Shelp, 89–103. Boston: D. Reidel, 1983.

21. Veatch, Robert M. "The Case for Contract in Medical Ethics." In *The Clinical Encounter*, edited by Earl E. Shelp, 105–12. Boston: D. Reidel, 1983.

22. Pellegrino, Edmund D. "The Anatomy of Clinical Judgments: Some Notes on Right Reason and Right Action." In *Clinical Judgment: A Critical Appraisal*, edited by H. Tristram Engelhardt, Jr., Stuart F. Spicker, and Bernard Towers, 169–94. Boston: D. Reidel, 1979.

23. Martin, Richard M. "A Clinical Model for Decision-Making." *Journal of Medical Ethics* 4 (1978): 200–206.

24. Jonsen, Siegler, and Winslade, *Clinical Ethics*.

25. Siegler, Mark. "Decision-Making Strategy for Clinical-Ethical Problems in Medicine." *Archives of Internal Medicine* 142 (1982): 2178–79.

26. Cassell, Eric J. "Clinical Practice, Clinical Ethics." *Archives of Internal Medicine* 145 (1985): 627–28.

27. Thomasma, David C. "Training in Medical Ethics: An Ethical Workup." *Forum on Medicine* 1 (1978): 33–36.

28. Pellegrino, Edmund D. "Humanistic Base for Professional Ethics in Medicine." *New York State Journal of Medicine* 77 (1977): 1456–62.

29. Sheldon, Gerald P. "Valedictory for Medical Residents." *Forum on Medicine* 1 (1978): 14–15.

30. Callahan, Daniel. "The Ethics Backlash." *Hastings Center Report* 5 (1975): 18.

31. Caplan, Arthur. "Applying Morality to Advances in Biomedicine: Can and Should This Be Done?" In *New Knowledge in the Biomedical Sciences*, edited by William B. Bondeson, H. Tristram Engelhardt, Jr., Stuart F. Spicker, and Joseph M. White, 155–68. Boston: D. Reidel, 1982.

32. Clouser, K. Danner. "Medical Ethics: Some Uses, Abuses and Limitations." *New England Journal of Medicine* 293 (1975): 384–87.

33. Swales, J. D. "Medical Ethics: Some Reservations." *Journal of Medical Ethics* 8 (1982): 117–19, 127.

34. Arras, John D., and Murray, Thomas H. "In Defence of Clinical Bioethics." *Journal of Medical Ethics* 8 (1982): 122–27.

35. Ruddick, William, and Finn, William. "Objections to Hospital Philosophers." *Journal of Medical Ethics* 11 (1985): 42–46.

36. Veatch, Robert M., and Sollitto, Sharmon. "Medical Ethics Teaching." *Journal of the American Medical Association* 235 (1976): 1030–33.

37. Ingelfinger, Franz J. "The Unethical in Medical Ethics." *Annals of Internal Medicine* 83 (1975): 264–69.

38. Churchill, Larry R. "Tacit Components of Medical Ethics: Making Decisions in the Clinic." *Journal of Medical Ethics* 3 (1977): 129–32.

39. Jonsen, Albert R. "Ethics as Immunotherapy." *Forum on Medicine* 1 (1978): 50–52.

40. Siegler, Mark. "A Legacy of Osler: Teaching Clinical Ethics at the Bedside." *Journal of the American Medical Association* 239 (1978): 951–56.

41. Thomasma, David C. "A Philosophy of Clinically Based Medical Ethics." *Journal of Medical Ethics* 6 (1980): 190-96.
42. Jonsen, Albert R. "Can an Ethicist Be a Consultant?" In *Frontiers in Medical Ethics*, edited by Virginia Abernethy, 157-71. Cambridge, MA: Ballinger, 1980.
43. Cassell, "Clinical Practice, Clinical Ethics."
44. Drane, James F. "Should a Hospital Ethicist Have Clinical Experience?" *Health Progress* 6 (1985): 60-63.
45. Hiatt, Howard H. "The Responsibilities of the Physician as a Member of Society: The Invisible Line." *Journal of Medical Education* 51 (1976): 30-38.
46. Ciccone, J. Richard, and Clements, Colleen. "Forensic Psychiatry and Applied Clinical Ethics: Theory and Practice." *American Journal of Psychiatry* 141 (1984): 395-99.
47. Clements, Colleen D., and Ciccone, J. Richard. "Applied Clinical Ethics or Universal Principles." *Hospital and Community Psychiatry* 36 (1985): 121-23.
48. Weinstein, Henry C. "Psychiatry on Trial: Clinical and Ethical Problems in Psychiatric Assessment of Competency to Stand Trial." *Annals of the New York Academy of Sciences* 347 (1980): 12-19.
49. Libow, Leslie S. "The Interface of Clinical and Ethical Decisions in the Care of the Elderly." *Mount Sinai Journal of Medicine* 48 (1981): 480-88.
50. Veatch, Robert M. "Defining the Techniques of an Experimental Program." In *The Teaching of Medical Ethics*, edited by Robert M. Veatch, Willard Gaylin, and Councilman Morgan, 61-65. Hastings-on-Hudson, NY: The Hastings Center, 1973.
51. Ruddick, William. "Can Doctors and Philosophers Work Together?" *Hastings Center Report* 11 (1981): 12-17.
52. Siegler, Mark; Rezler, Agnes G.; and Connell, Karen J. "Using Simulated Case Studies to Evaluate a Clinical Ethics Course for Junior Students." *Journal of Medical Education* 57 (1982): 380-85.
53. Thomasma, "A Philosophy of Clinically Based Medical Ethics."
54. Veatch, "Defining the Techniques of an Experimental Program."
55. Pellegrino, Edmund D. "Ethics and the Moment of Clinical Truth." *Journal of the American Medical Association* 239 (1978): 960-61.
56. Fleischman, Alan R. "A Physician's View." *Hastings Center Report* 11 (1981): 18-19.
57. Clouser, K. Danner. *Teaching Bioethics: Strategies, Problems, and Resources.* Hastings-on-Hudson, NY: The Hastings Center, 1980.
58. Ruddick, "Can Doctors and Philosophers Work Together?"

59. Pellegrino, "Ethics and the Moment of Clinical Truth."
60. Siegler, Mark. "Cautionary Advice for Humanists." *Hastings Center Report* 11 (1981): 19–20.
61. Fletcher, John C. "Who Should Teach Medical Ethics?" In *The Teaching of Medical Ethics*, edited by Robert M. Veatch, Willard Gaylin, and Councilman Morgan, 166–72. Hastings-on-Hudson, NY: The Hastings Center, 1973.
62. Siegler, "A Legacy of Osler: Teaching Clinical Ethics at the Bedside."
63. Dyck, Arthur J. *On Human Care: An Introduction to Ethics*. Nashville: Abingdon Press, 1977.

2

Conceptualizing the Role of the Ethics Consultant: Some Theoretical Issues

Terrence F. Ackerman

Ethics consultation is a genus which encompasses a variety of species. Its taxonomy can be developed through the use of appropriate interrogatives. For example, to whom are ethics consultations given? Possible recipients include patients, families, physicians, nurses, health care institutions, and government agencies. By whom are ethics consultations given? Providers might be individual ethicists, interdisciplinary teams, or ethics committees. About what are ethics consultations given? The focus might involve clinical care for individual patients or the development of research protocols, hospital regulations, or government policies.

Taxonomy is important because the properties that should characterize one species of ethics consultant may not characterize another. For example, we might maintain that ethics committees should not usurp the decision-making prerogatives of patients and physicians by making specific recommendations regarding clinical care, while holding that individual ethicists assisting in the formulation of government policies may offer specific policy proposals. Alternatively, it might be claimed that general properties can be identified that should apply to all types of consultation.

This chapter is devoted to one species of ethics consultant: the individual ethicist providing consultation to an attending physician regarding the care of a particular patient. Evidence suggests that this is the most frequently utilized form of ethics consultation.[1] The reader may consider whether the conclusions regarding this species are generalizable to other forms of ethics consultation.

This discussion includes four components: (1) description of the unique general function of an ethics consultant, (2) examination of key issues regarding the specific responsibilities of this role in consultations about the care of individual patients, (3) an outline of the features of moral inquiry and consideration of how they elucidate the appropriate ways to resolve these issues, and (4) a review of assumptions made in this analysis about the properties of moral reflection and about the societal needs that might be satisfied by institutionalizing the activity of ethics consultation.

THE GENERAL FUNCTION OF THE ETHICS CONSULTANT

A description of the general function of an ethics consultant begins with a consideration of the circumstances in which a physician might request assistance. This occurs when a clinical decision requires weighing of nontechnical value factors, and the physician is not readily able to utilize the conceptual tools (e.g., moral 'principles and their constituent concepts) or to secure the factual data (e.g., information regarding government regulations) that contribute to its reflective resolution. Assistance is requested that will lead the process of moral reflection to a satisfactory conclusion. Thus, as a preliminary hypothesis, we may propose that the general function of the ethics consultant should be to *facilitate* moral reflection or inquiry.

There are at least two kinds of situations that are commonly characterized as "moral problems." The type that is appropriately addressed in ethics consultation involves moral inquiry or reflection to determine which values or norms should be given priority in clinical caregiving. Another type of moral problem occurs when the appropriate goal or norm is recognized, but the conditions do not exist to make it a reality. The latter type has several species, such as situations in which the principal agent intentionally engages in morally wrong behavior (e.g., cheating on claims for insurance reimbursement), the attitudinal willingness to engage in correct behavior is weak (e.g., the exhausted resident cannot bring herself to discuss alternative treatment options with the patient), or the material resources are not available to achieve a recognized moral goal (e.g., a child's family does not have the money to purchase antibiotics needed for her recurrent kidney infections). This type of moral problem requires treatment by strategies other than moral reflection. The distinction is clinically important because the ethics consultant may sometimes be asked to deal with situations that are specific to the second kind of moral problem. But the ethics consultant has no special skills for resolving these problems, which may require such diverse actions as professional censure, changes in the conditions of professional training, or alterations in government assistance for indigent patients.

Although ethics consultants have the task of facilitating moral reflection, this is not all they do when providing consultations. Ethics consultants sometimes arbitrate between contending parties, provide emotional support for health professionals and patients, and offer spiritual guidance to persons seeking meaning in their suffering. Indeed, some ethics consultants (especially those with chaplaincy and/or counseling training) have degrees or training certificates (or both) that give official sanction for these activities. However, none of these activities uniquely characterizes ethics consultation. Its distinctive feature is the consultant's role as a facilitator of moral reflection, but much remains to be settled about the specifics of the consulting role.

QUESTIONS ABOUT THE CONSULTING ROLE

ANALYSIS VERSUS ANSWERS

One of the basic issues in defining the consulting role is whether ethics consultants should deliver "right" answers to the moral quandaries of physicians or should restrict their contribution to an analysis of the moral issues raised by particular cases.

Some theorists have maintained that bioethics will have significant social usefulness only if it permits the formulation of determinate solutions to moral quandaries in clinical medicine. For example, Callahan maintains that one criterion of good bioethical methodology should be that "it enables those who employ it to reach reasonably specific, clear decisions in those instances which require them — in the case of what is to be done about Mrs. Jones by four o'clock tomorrow afternoon, after which she will either live or die depending upon the decision made."[2] In a practical vein, Brody notes that the utility of a medical consultant is "based on his willingness to answer a very specific question which arises out of a complex practical problem in clinical medicine." Consequently, "the clinical consultant who advertises in advance that he will not give answers can be guaranteed a great deal of leisure time and relatively few consultations."[3]

The more modest role of analyst has been well articulated. It includes identifying the values or norms applicable to the case, clarifying the meaning of the principles and their constituent concepts, spelling out optional strategies for resolving the problem, and examining the concordance of the possible solutions with alternative views about priorities among principles. These activities are the traditional bread and butter of analytic philosophers.

Commentators have identified normative theoretical and moral reasons for restricting the consultant's role to analytic tasks. Nielsen's comprehensive review of normative ethical theory leads inexorably to the conclusion that "it is not clear what, if anything, could count as a foundation for morality, moral truth (true fundamental moral propositions) or a systematic knowledge of good and evil."[4] In the absence of such knowledge, Nielsen insists that there is no system of overarching principles from which we can derive solutions to concrete moral dilemmas. In addition, Morreim suggests that there are moral reasons for the consultant to avoid recommendations and to emphasize the process of moral reasoning. This emphasis will make physicians more adept at reaching consistently good decisions and will secure their acknowledgment that moral issues are supremely important and demand their thorough reflective consideration.[5]

REFLECTION VERSUS ACTION

Another fundamental issue concerns the role of the ethics consultant in implementing the solution that results from the consultative process. On one hand, we might maintain that the primary role of the consulting ethicist is to enrich, in cognitively useful ways, the moral reflection of the attending physician. If this approach is adopted, then the ethicist's primary obligation is complete after he or she skillfully utilizes philosophical methods to analyze the moral parameters of a case or to construct a recommendation for its resolution.

This approach produces an understanding of the ethicist's role that may differ significantly from the usual understanding of the physician's role. The physician's participation in a therapeutic relationship involves the commitment to serve the moral interests of the patient.[6] Failure to implement clinical care that is consistent with these interests violates a basic obligation. By contrast, the proposed understanding of the ethics consultant's role carries no obligation to assure that the moral interests of the patient are actually respected.

On the other hand, we might insist that an ethics consultant carries the obligation to assure that the solution that optimally protects the patient's moral interests (or those of other relevant parties) is actually adopted. If this approach is accepted, then the consulting ethicist must monitor the extent to which the solution has been implemented. Moreover, if there is a difference between the identified solution and the clinical care that is implemented, and if it significantly compromises the moral interests of the patient, then the ethics consultant will be obligated to seek appropriate revisions. This may entail additional discussions with the physician, patient, family members, or administrative officials. Thus, as protector of the patient's moral interests, the ethics consultant might enrich the moral reflection of the physician but also complicate his or her clinical management of the case.

ADVOCACY VERSUS IMPARTIALITY

An equally crucial question is whether the contribution of the ethics consultant should focus upon assessment of the moral interests of the patient or should embrace an impartial analysis of the competing moral interests of other relevant parties.

The standard view of the physician's role is that it includes an obligation to protect and promote the moral interests of the patient. There are recognized exceptions to this obligation. For example, the physician is generally thought to have a duty to break confidentiality when information revealed by the patient suggests that some other person has a high probability of being seriously and irreversibly harmed by the patient unless notified of the danger. But aside from a few carefully articulated exceptions, the duty to serve the patient's moral interests is assigned overriding weight. The same obligation devolves upon the medical consultant who enters a case at the request of the attending physician. By analogy, it might appear self-evident that the ethics consultant's primary obligation is to articulate and defend the patient's moral interests.

However, there are many moral problems in clinical medicine characterized by a conflict between the moral interests of the patient and those of other patients, family members, or society at large. For example, should the physician strongly encourage an unwilling but debilitated elderly patient to enter a nursing home, since he or she knows that the demands of care are causing a heavy physical and emotional burden for the daughter with whom the patient is living? Should the physician briefly sustain the life of a young child grievously injured in an auto accident until the parents can better accept the child's impending death? There is no a priori reason for assuming that the result of thorough moral reflection should always be assignment of priority status to the patient's moral interests. If the consultant's primary role is to skillfully facilitate moral reflection, it is possible that the analysis or recommendation may produce a clinical care plan that does not give preeminent weight to the patient's moral interests.

This possibility complicates our understanding of the

authorization permitting the physician to consult an ethicist. Transmission of privileged information regarding the patient is a standard feature of consultation. This is usually not problematic, since the moral bond between the attending physician and the patient carries the implicit agreement to draw upon institutional resources (including other health professionals) that may enhance the achievement of therapeutic goals. However, if the ethics consultant provides an analysis or recommendation that does not give priority to the patient's moral interests, it is not clear how his or her authorization to receive privileged information could derive from the tacit agreement of physician and patient regarding the terms of their relationship.

CRITIQUE VERSUS INTERPRETATION

Although a request for an ethics consultation usually means that a physician is not clear about his or her moral obligations in a specific clinical situation, various social factors may set de facto limits upon the options considered. First, there may be requirements of statute law, judicial precedents, or government regulations. The so-called Baby Doe regulations issued by the Department of Health and Human Services provide a well-known example. Second, there are moral principles and rules commonly acknowledged in the literature of medicine and medical ethics. One is the right of competent adult patients to refuse treatment. Third, social organizations within which ethics consultants work typically embody a set of implicit and explicit moral assumptions. These include the prevailing ethos (e.g., the "research imperative" at academic medical centers), the systematic theology or moral philosophy underlying some institutions (e.g., Catholic or Jewish hospitals), and existing policy guidelines for medical staff members (e.g., hospital rules regarding do-not-resuscitate orders).

An important issue is whether the content of the consulting ethicist's analysis or recommendations should be limited by these factors. On one hand, the ethics consultant is usually a salaried member of the institution. As a licensed and accredited facility, the hospital pledges to adhere to existing social norms (including legal rules) and formulates policy guidelines for implementing these norms under local conditions. In accepting a salaried position, any regular staff person seems to incur an obligation to function within the framework of social rules acknowledged by the institution. This commitment applies to members of the medical staff and might be extended to include the ethics consultant. If this line of reasoning is sound, then it appears that the consulting ethicist must constrain his or her analysis or recommendation within existing social parameters.

On the other hand, as an investigator of moral problems, the integrity of the ethics consultant's role seems to depend upon the freedom to frame whatever analyses or recommendations regarding the subject matter investigated are warranted by sound application of the methodology of the discipline. Moreover, it is obvious that existing laws, social norms, and institutional guidelines are often deficient from the standpoint of various moral parameters. Thus, there is the obvious possibility that the soundest advice that the ethics consultant can formulate may run contrary to the prevailing social norms under which a health care institution operates.

MORAL INQUIRY AND THE CONSULTATIVE PROCESS

These dilemmas arise when we attempt to clarify the details of the ethics consultant's role as a facilitator of moral reflection. In order to resolve them, we must first examine the nature of moral problems and the reflective process by which they are investigated.

Moral problems in medicine have these salient features: (1) it is difficult to identify patterns of interaction to which a shared commitment can be made; (2) general moral principles, based on past moral experience (such as respect for autonomy or concern for the well-being of others), suggest different patterns of interaction that might be instituted; and (3) there is an initial lack of social consensus regarding the appropriate pattern of social interaction.

Moral inquiry in medicine, the reflective process used to investigate such problems, includes the following properties:

1. Moral inquiry is a process that seeks plans of action evoking a *shared social commitment* among members of the moral community. Moral problems involve situations in which there is a lack of social agreement regarding the appropriate pattern of behavior. Consequently, their resolution involves a broadening of our common moral bonds.

2. There is an irreducible element of *human choice* in the resolution of these moral problems. Moral reflection involves identification of patterns of social interaction that will make secure the diverse states of affairs cherished by different members of the moral community. Consequently, the content of what is morally obligatory, permissible, and so on, depends upon what is cherished. Rachels captures this point succinctly when he writes that "ethics provides answers about what we ought to do, given that we are the kinds of creatures we are, caring about the things we will care about when we are as reasonable as we can be, living in the sort of circumstances in which we live."[7]

3. Plans of action are sought that will *impartially* recognize the diverse activities cherished by different members of the moral community. For example, dying patients may prefer quite different styles or modes of dying. Alternative forms of social interaction may be more or less supportive of the activities persons cherish. Thus, moral inquiry seeks plans that respect the diversity of things cherished by different persons.

4. Alternative plans for resolving moral problems typically reflect different valued features of social interaction (such as not interfering with other persons or contributing to the enhancement of their well-being). Often these valued features of social interaction cannot be simultaneously endorsed. Consequently, moral reflection seeks a shared *setting of priorities*.

5. Moral inquiry seeks plans of action that will be *reflectively* accepted by members of the moral community. Plans of action must operate and have their consequences in the real world. The objective of moral reflection is not mere social agreement but an agreement that can be sustained because, in actual operation, the plan promotes the outcomes cherished by diverse members of the moral community. Thus, the consensus must be molded by persons who are thoroughly familiar with relevant values, facts, options, and the consequences of their implementation.

6. When a member of the moral community proposes a solution to a moral problem, he or she is proposing a *hypothesis*. The hypothesis is that the plan of action will actually support the diverse activities cherished by different members of the moral community and will therefore sustain a shared social commitment. Verification of the hypothesis depends upon reflective confirmation by other members of the moral community that the plan of action does, in fact, respect the states of affairs that they deem worthy of realization.

These features of moral inquiry carry implications for the resolution of the issues raised regarding the role of the ethics consultant. First, the ethics consultant cannot and should not provide all the answers. The goal of moral inquiry is to develop plans for dealing with morally problematic situations in a way that will evoke shared social commitments. Therefore, morally appropriate behavior cannot be determined without the input of other members of the moral community who participate in the reflective process. In this respect, the justification of moral claims closely parallels the process by which scientific claims gain status. The latter achieve justification only when different investigators arrive at similar conclusions by following similar procedures in dealing with the problematic subject matter. Since justified moral commitments are socially produced outcomes, the ethicist cannot know what is right independently of the reflective contribution of other members of the moral community.

Recommendations by the ethics consultant are not ruled out, but the consulting ethicist must clearly convey the *status* of the recommendation. It is not an assertion that a particular course of action has been independently determined to be the morally correct option. Rather, the recommendation is a hypothesis that a particular plan of action will be endorsed by other members of the moral community because it will be effective in promoting the states of affairs they cherish. Thus, it cannot be accepted independently of the confirmatory reflection and experience of the health professionals consulted.

Second, the ethics consultant should not be viewed as a monitor of the clinical care received by the patient. Assignment of this role assumes that the ethics consultant has special access to knowledge regarding the patient's moral interests. However, the process of moral inquiry suggests that obligations toward the patient must be determined in a reflective social dialogue. While the ethics consultant may possess certain knowledge and skills necessary to facilitate this reflective process, he or she does not have access to the solution to the moral problem. Therefore, there are no strong grounds for assigning to the ethics consultant a special role in monitoring the patient's clinical care.

Public discussion of moral issues in medicine—in newspaper columns, TV broadcasts, academic journals, and scholarly books—is part of the social process of moral inquiry described above. A good ethics consultant should be intimately familiar with the reflective consensus that often emerges from this public dialogue. Insofar as he or she is knowledgeable about the consensus that has tentatively formed, this information can be conveyed to the attending physician. Nevertheless, this tentative consensus is still subject to the confirmatory reflection of the health professionals consulted.

This position does not absolve the consulting ethicist of an obligation to "blow the whistle" on clearly immoral behavior in the clinical care of patients. However, we must keep in mind the distinction between the main types of moral problems.

Ethics consultation is appropriate to situations in which it is unclear which human values should take priority and which clinical care option should be implemented. Sometimes even conscientious moral agents cannot reach a reflective consensus about the appropriate resolution to a clinical moral problem. But these are not the paradigmatic situations generating an obligation to "blow the whistle." Whistle blowing is most appropriate in situations where certain behaviors are obviously wrong. Therefore, no special obligations devolve upon the ethics consultant in his or her specific role, since facilitation of moral inquiry involves situations in which the morally appropriate course of action is not obvious. However, a general obligation to report wrong behavior applies to any moral agent in a position to spot behavior that is seriously wrong from a legal or moral standpoint.

Third, the ethics consultant must impartially represent the moral interests of all relevant parties. The function of moral inquiry is to identify patterns of social interaction that evoke a shared social commitment, because they impartially protect and promote the diverse outcomes cherished by different members of the moral community. As a facilitator of moral reflection, the ethics consultant has a responsibility to assure that the variety of moral interests relevant to a situation are fully considered in constructing a solution. The locus of these moral interests does not reside exclusively with the patient, nor do the interests of the patient always achieve priority status in moral inquiry. Therefore, the ethics consultant cannot be considered only an advocate for the moral interests of the patient without jeopardizing the integrity of the reflective process.

However, if the ethics consultant is not committed to serve only the moral interests of the patient, it appears that his or her authorization cannot be derived from the authorization given by the patient to the attending physician. There are two ways to resolve this dilemma: First, we might admit that the original commitment of the physician is limited to protecting only those moral interests of the patient that retain priority status when in conflict with the moral interests of other relevant parties. This strategy appears quite reasonable, since there are already recognized exceptions (such as those regarding confidentiality) which limit obligations to the patient. If the original commitment of the physician is limited, then the authorization which the ethics consultant derives from that agreement might be similarly limited. Second, we might identify a source of authorization for the ethics consultant other than the initial agreement between physician and patient. For example, the consultant's authorization to review confidential case material might be compared to that of "quality control" functionaries in the administrative apparatus of health care facilities. These functionaries, such as peer review officials, have authorization to review case material with regard to social objectives (such as cost containment) not directly related to the well-being or other moral interests of particular patients. In the case of the ethics consultant, the quality control function might be to assure that the moral interests of all relevant parties are properly considered in clinical decision making.

Fourth, the role of the ethics consultant should be constructed, from an organizational standpoint, in a way that permits maximum investigative freedom to critically assess existing social rules related to the care of patients. There are at least two reasons. First, legal rules and institutional policies are intended to promote specific states of affairs cherished by members of the moral community. However, they are often unlikely to represent other states of affairs that members of the moral community also regard as worthy. Assignment of a critical function to the ethics consultant helps to assure the impartial review of relevant moral considerations essential to competent moral inquiry. Second, legal rules and institutional guidelines may be developed under conditions that do not fully satisfy the requirements of rigorous moral inquiry. Thorough reflection involves determining whether options adopted are effective in protecting states of affairs cherished by members of the moral community. Building justification for our moral decisions (as embodied in legal and institutional rules) depends upon critical examination of how these guidelines work out in a variety of clinical circumstances. Assigning to ethics consultants a critical (versus merely interpretive) function permits thorough review of the clinical operation of existing social rules. Thus, a critical role for ethics consultants may enhance the development of shared social norms, the commitment to which is sustained by their development according to rigorous methods of moral reflection.

Of course, consultative analysis or advice that is inconsistent with existing legal or institutional rules may be more difficult to justify. Insofar as these rules have been formulated through formal social mechanisms (undergoing legislative approval or administrative review within a health care institution), their development may reflect a social consensus built upon careful assessment of relevant values, options, and the consequences of their implementation. Moreover, acceptance of existing social rules promotes rule-observing behavior in general and respect for the formal mechanisms by which rules are developed. Nevertheless, the general social benefits of open inquiry also have been powerfully articulated in the literature of moral and political philosophy.[8]

Assumptions Underlying the Analysis

The foregoing analysis of the consulting role is dependent upon various assumptions. If these assumptions were altered, we would be likely to adopt a significantly different formulation of the role of the ethics consultant. The assumptions are of two main types.

First, there are assumptions about the purpose and procedures of moral inquiry. The earlier description maintains that "right answers" to moral issues are shared social commitments, dependent upon human choice and determinable in a reflective and experimental social process. By contrast, one might argue that there are truths about our moral obligations, independent of human choice and discoverable by special methods of philosophical reasoning. The latter assumptions would alter the conclusions in at least a couple of ways. It would be reasonable to assign to the ethics consultant a responsibility for determining the right answers to moral dilemmas in clinical care. Moreover, if the ethics consultant has special access to moral knowledge, then it seems reasonable to require that ethics consultants monitor the extent to which the patient's clinical care conforms to the dictates of this moral truth.

Second, there are assumptions about the specific social problems that generate the need for ethics consultations and that might be ameliorated by institutionalizing the consulting role. The previous analysis deals with situations in which physicians are uncertain about which values or norms should be endorsed and implemented. Facilitation of moral inquiry provides cognitive assistance to physicians in determining which setting of priorities and plan for clinical care might secure a shared social commitment. Thus, both the social problems and their solution are assumed to be cognitive in nature. By contrast, one might argue that the most serious moral problems arising in the clinical care of patients involve the failure of physicians to respect publicly recognized moral rules regulating therapeutic interaction. If this premise is accepted, then it might be appropriate to assign to ethics consultants a responsibility for monitoring clinical care plans actually implemented. Moreover, if the failure to respect the moral interests of patients is the most common violation of acknowledged moral rules, the role of the ethics consultant might be restricted to protecting the moral interests of patients. These role responsibilities would help reduce the incidence of violations of publicly acknowledged moral rules in therapeutic encounters.

Thus, the foregoing conceptualization of the role of the ethics consultant depends heavily upon the theory of moral reflection presented and the social problems identified as the appropriate subject matter for the consultant's activities.

NOTES

1. See Appendix: A Survey of Ethics Consultants.
2. Daniel Callahan, "Bioethics as a Discipline," *Hastings Center Studies* 1 (1973): 66–73.
3. Howard Brody, "Teaching Clinical Ethics: Models for Consideration," in *Clinical Medical Ethics: Exploration and Assessment*, ed. Terrence F. Ackerman, Glenn C. Graber, Charles H. Reynolds, and

David C. Thomasma (Lanham, MD: University Press of America, 1987), pp. 31–42.

4. Kai Nielsen, "On Being Skeptical about Applied Ethics," in *Clinical Medical Ethics: Exploration and Assessment*, ed. Terrence F. Ackerman, Glenn C. Graber, Charles H. Reynolds, and David C. Thomasma (Lanham, MD: University Press of America, 1987), pp. 95–115.

5. E. Haavi Morreim, "The Philosopher in the Clinical Setting," *Pharos* 46 (1983): 2–6.

6. The phrase "moral interests" includes all behavior by other persons that an individual can expect from them as a matter of moral obligation. The patient's moral interests include the opportunity to give informed consent to treatment, to reveal personal information in confidence, and to receive competent medical care. Thus, moral interests include more than physician behavior that promotes the patient's welfare.

7. James Rachels, "Can Ethics Provide Answers?" *Hastings Center Report* 10 (1980): 32–40.

8. John Stuart Mill, *On Liberty* (Indianapolis: Bobbs-Merrill, 1956).

3

Ethics in the Clinical Setting

Joy D. Skeel and Donnie J. Self

Ethics has always been important in the practice of medicine. For centuries, medical ethics has been informally taught through role modeling and publicly endorsed through various medical codes of ethics. The last two decades, however, have brought increasing interest in ethics in medicine, as evidenced by the development of an enormous body of academic literature and a specialized discipline of trained professionals who grapple with issues in medical ethics. The popular press has covered this development for lay persons. Much of this interest in medical ethics has been manifested in the development of formal courses in medical ethics, which are taught at both the undergraduate and medical school levels. Although the exact number of medical ethics courses that are now being taught at the undergraduate level is not known, such courses have become very popular in colleges and universities across the country. Clear documentation is available at the medical school level. Pellegrino and McElhinney report that the number of U.S. medical schools that include medical ethics in their required curricula rose from 4.2 percent in 1972 to 72.8 percent in 1982.[1] Almost all medical schools now offer some course in medical ethics. Indeed, medical ethics is not a fad; it has become firmly entrenched in medical school curricula.

Attention has now turned to the teaching of ethics in residency training.[2-7] The Society for Health and Human Values recently reported the results of a special project analyzing the status of ethics teaching in primary care residency training.[8] An interest group within the society will continue to pursue these issues. Other professional organizations that have developed task forces to address the teaching of ethics in residency training include the Society of Teachers of Family Medicine, the American Board of Internal Medicine, the Ambulatory Pediatrics Association, and the Society for Research and Education in Primary Care Internal Medicine. For several years, these groups have vigorously pursued the goal of incorporating ethics teaching into residency training.

Interest is focused not only on the teaching of ethics in medical training but also on the implementation of ethical concepts in medical practice.[9,10] This is evidenced by the growing attention to and utilization of ethics consultations in clinical medicine as well as the enormous increase in interest in hospital ethics committees.[11-13] The increased interest is partly a response to publicity surrounding Quinlan, Conroy, Baby Doe, and other such cases. It has been suggested that increased attention to clinical ethics is merely an example of "defensive medicine," a means by which physicians minimize the possibility of complicated legal entanglements. But whatever the reasons, the ethical aspects of the practice of medicine are being given more explicit and formal attention. This has resulted in an enormous increase in the number of ethicists, or people with at least some formal training in and exposure to ethics, who function as consultants in the clinical setting.

In talking with our colleagues around the country, we sensed a heightened level of clinical concern and activity in medical ethics from people with secular as well as religious backgrounds in ethics. We began to analyze the different roles that our ethicist colleagues filled in clinical settings, noting that they fell into four categories of activities. We then began to think about the conceptual issues involved in the various categories and subsequently developed four hypothetical roles for the ethicist in the clinical setting. These roles, which have been described in detail elsewhere,[14] are briefly outlined below.

The first role concerns the medical ethicist who is called in to make recommendations on patient care in difficult cases. This model involves the ethicist in active and direct aspects of patient care. The ethicist is viewed as a professional who has special expertise (presumably in ethical decision making) and who sees patients, collects and processes data, and then assists the physician in making difficult decisions about the patient's care. Of course, as with other medical and surgical consultants, the ethicist can make probability statements but cannot provide definitive answers to complex questions.

A second interpretation of the role of the ethicist in the clinical setting is that of an educator who works with health care providers, students, and staff (but usually not with patients) to analyze issues and raise questions, but does not attempt or claim to dispense answers to complex questions. It is sufficient for the ethicist to illuminate connections, enumerate options, clarify reasoning, define the boundaries of concepts, and point out presuppositions. This results in increased sensitivity and greater open-mindedness and encourages an attitude of conceptual excitement in the practice of medicine. Here the ethicist possesses a different kind of expertise, namely the ability to analyze concepts and illuminate issues. In this model, the ethicist is involved only in passive and indirect aspects of patient care, and may or may not actively see patients in order to accomplish the necessary objectives. The ethicist is more concerned with illuminating generalizable features concerning certain types of cases than with determining what to do in a particular case, although direct action may in fact result from clarification of an issue with generalizable features.

A third role for the ethicist in the clinical setting is that of a counselor to health care providers (medical students, residents, attendings, and staff) but not to patients. The ethicist is not expected to function as a psychotherapist or even as a formal counselor of any sort but as a kind of catharsis worker, allowing health care providers to unburden themselves to someone who will simply reflect and accept their statements without passing judgment. This is particularly helpful when a health care provider has made an error and needs reassurance and moral support; medical ethicists are frequently sought out for this purpose. However, the role of counselor is certainly not limited to cases of error or even solely to professional issues.

Health care providers frequently turn to medical ethicists for help with personal problems. In the role of counselor, the medical ethicist is not directly involved in patient care. Of course, patient care is indirectly influenced by the health of the caregiver.

Finally, the patient advocate model depicts the ethicist as one who protects patients and defends their rights. The ethicist assists patients in maintaining their autonomy, especially with regard to informed consent. Here the ethicist assists the patient rather than the physician in decision making. The ethicist generally looks out for the patient's best interest and, in so doing, is actively involved in patient care. The medical ethicist presumably has expertise (objectivity or disinterest, as opposed to lack of interest) and the ability to provide conceptual clarity in dealing with complex issues. If not performed carefully, this role may put the ethicist in an adversarial position in relation to the physician.

After developing this theoretical scheme, we collected empirical data on how ethicists actually function in the clinical setting. Three questionnaires were developed to obtain information from several sources about who functions as an ethicist in the clinical (i.e., hospital or clinic) setting, what role they most frequently perform (i.e., consultant, educator, counselor, or patient advocate), and which of the four models the respondents thought would be most helpful to physicians. The three questionnaires were sent to hospital chaplains, medical ethicists, and physicians, respectively.

The demographic questions, regarding the location of the respondent's institution, gender, and age, were the same on all questionnaires. The questionnaire to chaplains and medical ethicists asked about educational background and whether they were involved in clinical activity as medical ethicists, as well as what percentage of their time was spent in that role. Physicians were asked about their area of specialization. Chaplains and medical ethicists were requested to indicate on a scale of 1 to 5 how often they functioned in the role of consultant, educator, counselor, or patient advocate, and to note which of these roles they regarded as most helpful to physicians. The final part of the questionnaire asked whether the respondent (1) taught via conferences for physicians, medical students, and nurses; (2) participated in medical teaching rounds at the bedside; and (3) provided ethics consultations for specific patients. If they provided consultations, they were asked whether they made recommendations regarding patient care, made entries on the patient's chart, or charged a fee for such consultations.

The questionnaire to physicians asked about the educational backgrounds of medical ethics professionals working in the clinical setting in their institutions. Physicians were requested to indicate on a scale of 1 to 5 how often the medical ethics professional functioned as a consultant, educator, counselor, or patient advocate and which of the four models they found most helpful. Finally, they were asked to indicate how many consultations they had requested from the medical ethicist during the past year.

The questionnaires were distributed to the members of the Society for Health and Human Values and to member hospitals of the American Hospital Association with 200 or more beds. The questionnaires were approved for distribution by the American Hospital Association. Over 3,000 questionnaires were distributed and the response rate was surprising. Although a limited response was expected, well over 600 questionnaires were returned. Some hospital administrators wrote that their hospitals did not have a medical ethicist; others described their hospital ethics committees. Some respondents wrote notes or letters regarding their interest in the project and offering their support. The project is still underway, and preliminary analysis of the data has begun.

According to the early data, approximately 67 percent of those returning the medical ethicist questionnaire were involved in clinical activity. Fifty percent of the medical ethicist respondents said that they provided ethics consultations for specific patients, as opposed to performing rounds or providing teaching conferences.

Similarly, approximately 67 percent of chaplain respondents indicated that they were involved in clinical activity. However, 75 percent provide ethics consultations for specific patients; this may indicate that chaplains are more patient-oriented, whereas medical ethicists are more involved in staff educational activities.

Approximately 33 percent of physician respondents indicated that their institutions employed a medical ethics professional other than a chaplain.

These trends may not hold up after the entire body of data has been processed. Further analysis of the data will indicate the perceived usefulness of the four models of the medical ethicist as well as whether they make entries on patient charts, provide specific recommendations for patient care, and charge a fee for their services.

This is the beginning of a research project to gather empirical data on the work of clinical ethicists. Little such research has been reported in the literature of either medicine or ethics. The findings of this project will help to clarify the nature of the activities of the clinical ethicist.

REFERENCES

1. Pellegrino, Edmund D., and McElhinney, Thomas K. *Teaching Ethics, the Humanities and Human Values in Medical Schools: A Ten Year Overview*. Washington, DC: Society for Health and Human Values, 1982.
2. Self, Donnie J., and Lyon-Loftus, G. T. "A Model for Teaching Ethics in Family Medicine Residency." *Journal of Family Practice* 16 (1983): 355–59.
3. Sun, T., and Self, Donnie J. "Medical Ethics Programs in Family Practice Residencies." *Family Medicine* 17 (1985): 99–102.
4. Geyman, J. P. "Expanding Concerns and Applications of Medical Ethics." *Journal of Family Practice* 10 (1980): 595–96.
5. Dayringer, Richard; Paira, Rosalia E. A.; and Davidson, Glen W. "Ethical Decision Making by Family Physicians." *Journal of Family Practice* 17 (1983): 267–72.
6. Carson, Ronald A., and Curry, R. W., Jr. "Ethics Teaching on Ward Rounds." *Journal of Family Practice* 11 (1980): 59.
7. Brody, Howard. "The Current Status of Humanities in Family Medicine Education." *Family Medicine* 14 (1982): 3–8.
8. Society for Health and Human Values. *The Teaching of Humanities*

and Human Values in Primary Care Residency Training: Resource Book. McLean, VA: Society for Health and Human Values, 1984.

9. Perkins, Henry S., and Saatoff, B. S. "Do Ethics Consultations Help in Patient Care?" *Clinical Research* 34 (1986): 271A.

10. Purtilo, Ruth. "Ethics Consultations in the Hospital." *New England Journal of Medicine* 311 (1984): 983–86.

11. Levine, Carol. "Questions and Some Very Tentative Answers About Hospital Ethics Committees." *Hastings Center Report* 14 (1984): 9–12.

12. Youngner, Stuart J.; Jackson, David L.; Coulton, Claudia; Juk-nialis, Barbara W.; and Smith, Era M. "A National Survey of Hospital Ethics Committees." *Critical Care Medicine* 11 (1983): 902–5.

13. Cranford, Ronald E., and Doudera, A. Edward. "The Emergence of Institutional Ethics Committees." *Law, Medicine and Health Care* 12 (1984): 13–20.

14. Self, Donnie J., and Skeel, Joy D. "Potential Roles of the Medical Ethicist in the Clinical Setting." *Theoretical Medicine* 7 (1986): 33–39.

Part II

The Ethics Consultant in the Hospital

INTRODUCTION

Part II contains three chapters that discuss the role and functions of ethics consultants in hospitals and one chapter that advises hospitals on how to hire an ethicist. John C. Fletcher and Maxwell Boverman describe the evolution of the role of the bioethicist at the Warren G. Magnuson Clinical Center, National Institutes of Health (NIH), a 500-bed research hospital. Originally, physicians saw the ethicist as an adversary, to be consulted only after help was obtained from a psychiatric consultant. However, the ethicist's role gradually crystallized to include three functions: teacher, consultant, and bridge to authority. This chapter also claims that, in its effort to respond to ethical problems in research activities, the NIH added the role of a bioethicist as a source of protection for research subjects.

Ruth B. Purtilo, an ethics consultant in a teaching hospital, examines four models for consultation in order to gain perspective on the new enterprise: (1) clinical consultation as understood in medicine, (2) consultee-centered case consultation, (3) consultation as understood in commerce and business, and (4) consultation as understood by liaison-psychiatrists. She examines the strengths and weaknesses of each model.

Anne J. Davis is a nurse-ethicist often called in to mediate ethical disputes between nurses and physicians. Her chapter gives two case histories of such disputes. Since, at the time, her role as ethics consultant was not salaried or officially supported by the institution, there was plenty of potential for trouble. Yet, this situation exists today in many institutions where talented individuals provide consultation before the institution incorporates a role for the consultant.

James F. Drane addresses hospitals interested in hiring an ethicist and reviews the reasons that physicians and other hospital staff need training in ethics. Drane then considers the risks of hiring the wrong kind of ethicist: antimedical values, authoritarianism, and false conceptions of medicine. Administrators with the responsibility for creating a job description for a hospital ethicist and for interviewing candidates would be well advised to read Drane's discussion of the "right kind" of ethicist.

4

The Evolution of the Role of an Applied Bioethicist in a Research Hospital

John C. Fletcher and Maxwell Boverman

The Warren G. Magnuson Clinical Center (CC) is a 500-bed research hospital, opened in 1953 as the clinical arm of the National Institutes of Health (NIH). Almost all of the intramural clinical research of the NIH's ten institutes is conducted in the CC.[1] In 1986, the CC had 8,582 admissions and an average inpatient census of 350. Additionally, it housed 72 normal volunteers, mainly college students, who participated in studies while living and working as laboratory assistants for three or more months. Also, 3,726 normal volunteers from the surrounding community took part in studies but did not live in the CC. More than 1,000 physicians and scientists conduct clinical research in more than 1,000 research projects. Each patient volunteer is admitted under a "protocol," a written plan that details research activities and goals and includes a consent form.

Mortimer B. Lipsett, director of the CC (1976 to 1982), employed a bioethicist for the first time in August 1977. This chapter describes the evolution of the bioethicist's role in this research hospital since that time. It is based on the experience of the authors and on interviews with the director and former deputy director of the CC, several clinical directors (chief medical officers in the intramural program of the institutes), retired officials, and a study of relevant policy and historical documents. The questions posed in the interviews were (1) How did preexist-

ing conditions influence the decision to employ a bioethicist?
(2) How did the role of the bioethicist evolve? (3) What ethical
problems in clinical research does the bioethicist deal with at
present?

PREEXISTING CONDITIONS

Prior to World War II, scientists in the United States only
occasionally voiced concerns about the ethics of human experimentation. Their main concern was with the primitive state of
the law with respect to the differences between research and
practice, especially in medicine. Only one recorded prewar
court case, *Bonner* v. *Moran*, dealt with a specific dispute about
wrongdoing in research.[2] However, the trials of 23 German
physicians in 1946 for "war crimes and crimes against human-
ity" dramatically alerted medical and political leaders to a
need.[3] Medical research could greatly benefit society, but social
controls were needed to prevent harm done to human beings in
the name of the state or by unethical investigators. The Nuremberg Code set forth basic ethical principles to guide the
planning and conduct of medical research.[4] Although the
code's legal status was disputed, due to its origin in an international body, most of its substance was the moral core of all later
codes and expressions of research ethics. European medical
societies and the American Medical Association (AMA)
adopted the essentials of the code in the 1950s and 1960s.
Researchers at the NIH discussed the code's relevance to
research as the CC was being opened in the early 1950s.[5]

PRIOR GROUP REVIEW OF RISK AND BENEFIT

The historical origins of prior group review lie in the practice of
consultation between physicians and surgeons, before starting
innovative therapy, in major European hospitals during the
eighteenth and nineteenth centuries.[6] When the CC opened, a
document had been prepared requiring "group consideration"
of clinical research procedures that "deviated from acceptable
medical practice or involved unusual hazards."[7,8] A clinical

research committee (CRC) was organized as a subcommittee of the medical board of the CC to deliberate on scientific and ethical questions in research proposals referred to it by clinical directors, senior clinical investigators, and the office of the director of the NIH.

G. Burroughs Mider, the first chairman of the CRC, recalls that two of the first set of protocols for patient studies were disapproved (personal communication, April 30, 1982). An investigator proposed to leave indwelling intravascular catheters in patients to make continuous measurements. The procedure was considered too risky, because the catheters were breakable and were made of woven material. A proposed study involving needle biopsy of the liver in patients was also refused.

In 1954, the director of the NIH ordered the CRC to review all research involving newly arrived normal volunteers.[9] The office of the director exercised second-level review of normal volunteer studies. This extra precaution reflected a standard that research risks for normal persons had to be minimal. In 1961, the CRC was assigned review responsibility for all patient studies that were only investigative or "nontherapeutic" in purpose. In keeping with the older tradition of medicine, new therapeutic studies were discussed in formal and informal ward consultations between the principal investigator, senior physicians, and other interested colleagues.

In the 1950s and 1960s, research review was the major way that NIH researchers showed their ethical concern for the safety of research subjects. Research review was grafted onto older, more established ethical procedures that also applied to newer, more complex relationships of physician-investigator and subject. The welfare of the patient and the benefit of the scientific goal were the major ethical standards in the review process. Evidently, these efforts at the NIH were influential steps in the early evolution of research ethics. Two studies in the early 1960s showed that only 10 percent of university departments of medicine had research review bodies.[10,11] Further, these studies uncovered widespread skepticism among clinical researchers about the value of developing written guidelines for research. The ethics of research were still largely embedded in and undifferentiated from the ethics of medicine.[12]

FAMOUS CASES AND THEIR CONSEQUENCES

Some famous cases in the 1960s and early 1970s troubled the public reputation of clinical research and created a furor in the media, professional journals, and the U.S. Congress. Much of the discussion favored further social controls on research and the protection of human subjects.

1. In 1966, two well-known physicians in New York were suspended from the practice of medicine for one year after a dispute about the lack of informed consent in a study of the immune response. Live cancer cells were injected into chronically ill patients without disclosure, presumably in the interest of not frightening the patients.[13]

2. In 1966, Henry Beecher published a notable article with 22 examples of research he considered ethically questionable due to excessive risk or lack of informed consent.[14]

3. In 1966, researchers in an institution for retarded children were criticized for infecting children with hepatitis virus to study the period of infectivity prior to testing a vaccine.[15]

4. In 1972, it was revealed that scientists in the Public Health Service (PHS) had withheld therapy from black males with syphilis to study the natural history of the disease. The so-called Tuskegee experiment in rural Alabama had begun in 1932.[16,17]

5. In 1973, research with "live abortuses" caused a furor in Congress, and students of a nearby Catholic high school, led by Eunice Kennedy Shriver, visited the NIH to protest alleged research "funded by the NIH with live abortuses." NIH officials issued denials and stated their opposition to such research.[18]

Actual practices in these and a small number of other documented cases fell far short of the ideals in codes of ethics espoused by leaders in European and American medical research (e.g., the Declaration of Helsinki and the AMA code of ethics).[19] These revelations, and fear that there might be many more such abuses, led to a movement in the NIH and the PHS to find policy levers to protect human subjects. Simultaneously, the civil rights movement reinforced the awakening of interest in policy change among members of the federal research community. The development of powerful new drugs and tools, such as hemodialysis, organ transplantation, and the potential to manipulate the genetic code, created in many an urge for order in a swiftly changing and often morally bewildering sphere of social life. A movement for "bioethics" arose in the later 1960s and was marked by interdisciplinary and public debate about the proper uses of new biomedical technologies.[20]

Although none of these notorious cases arose in the NIH, the intensity of the congressional and media debate of the issues had an impact on NIH leaders. Veteran researchers recalled older experiments with patients and volunteers that were clearly unacceptable in the light of the newer standards of group review and informed consent. Prior to 1966, most consent practices were verbal in nature. Only surgery routinely involved written consent. Some CC researchers were convinced that interest in written consent documents only masked a "charade" to protect the institution from lawsuits.[21] Despite its share of skepticism, the NIH shaped effective policies to protect human subjects. NIH Director James Shannon was concerned about the scanty practices of prior group review in grantee institutions and provided steady leadership throughout this turbulent period.

GROWTH OF POLICIES AND PROCEDURES TO PROTECT HUMAN SUBJECTS

In February 1966, after extensive discussion in the PHS and the NIH, the surgeon general ordered that any institution funded by the PHS for research with human subjects was required to provide a prior institutional review of each project.[22] In 1971, the PHS policy was extended to all research conducted or supported by the Department of Health, Education, and Welfare (DHEW). Thereby, much more behavioral and social science research was brought under the policy.

Prior to 1966, NIH researchers themselves had changed intramural (CC) policy and procedures to ensure more protection of patients and normal volunteers. In 1964, an ad hoc committee was appointed by Jack Masur, director of the CC. The group was charged with evaluating the existing practices of group review and consent that had evolved since the 1953 document. Under the leadership of Nathaniel Berlin, clinical director of the National Cancer Institute (NCI), the committee conducted an in-depth study of the existing system of review by the medical board CRC, and interviewed each clinical director and many senior investigators about their practices in peer consultation prior to new trials of therapy with patients. Their recommendations for research review resulted in the formation of the CRC of the medical board.

ETHICS AT THE NIH

The new standards and practices developed at the NIH to protect human subjects have contributed to the development of research ethics throughout the nation. In 1966, John Fletcher began a research project at the CC to study the ethics of medical research.[23] He met, interviewed, and observed many of the researchers with whom he would later work as bioethicist. The term *bioethics* did not come into existence until the early 1970s, when it began to be used to describe ethical issues in the biomedical sciences.[24,25]

Robert Marston, director of the NIH from 1968 to 1973, discussed ethics in human research in a lecture delivered at the University of Virginia in 1972.[26] He was concerned about the extramural programs' responsibility to encourage high ethical standards. The Marston paper led to the appointment of an NIH (later PHS) committee to draft regulations for the protection of human subjects.[27] DHEW concurrently published proposed regulations for research with the human fetus and pregnant women. The DHEW committee, known as the "study group," was later chaired by Charles McCarthy and evolved into the PHS steering committee for the protection of human research subjects.

In 1974, the Institutional Relations Branch of NIH's Division of Research Grants, the unit responsible for the administration of DHEW policy on research protection, was transformed into the Office for Protection from Research Risks (OPRR). Today, OPRR administers Department of Health and Human Services (DHHS) policy for protection of human subjects and oversees the compliance of grantees with a requirement for a written "assurance" that all DHHS standards for the review process are met.

In the early 1970s, congressional discussion of some of the famous cases described above, under the leadership of Senator Edward Kennedy and Representative Paul Rogers, led to legislation that created the National Commission for the Protection of Human Subjects of Biomedical and Behavioral Research. The National Research Act, signed in July 1974 (Public Law 93-348, 88 Stat. 343, 42 U.S.C.), charged the 11-member body appointed by DHEW's secretary to identify the basic ethical principles that should underlie the conduct of human research. The commission was also mandated to study a variety of ethical questions about categories of vulnerable subjects (e.g., fetuses, children, the institutionalized mentally disabled, and prisoners). Thus, the ethical debate about principles and procedures in human research had penetrated to the center of public policymaking. Out of the debate came an even more impartial body to consider measures to regulate research. The law provided that the commission's recommendations would become DHHS policy unless the secretary published reasons why these would be inappropriate.

Two early recommendations made by the commission soon affected research review at the CC and elsewhere. In 1975, DHEW issued new regulations for institutional review boards (IRBs). Also, new definitions of standards for the process of consent by research subjects were released. Previously, the review body had only to assure that it documented the steps the researcher took to obtain informed consent.

These regulations coincided with a period of intense study of all CC policies and practices that affected the welfare of research subjects. When Donald Fredrickson became NIH director in 1974, his interest turned to the intramural research programs and the quality of patient care in the CC. He believed the CC to be central to the NIH's best contribution to clinical medicine. Under his leadership, a process of change began with another intense look at policies and practices that directly affected patients in research. Griff T. Ross, then a senior investigator at the National Institute of Child Health and Human Development (NICHHD), directed policy studies and the changes in bylaws and research review that followed.

These changes resulted in the centralization of all patient and normal volunteer research review in a two-level process.[28] The CRCs were renamed "institute clinical review subpanels" (ICRSs), and their memberships were enlarged for a richer interdisciplinary mix. The medical board was henceforth responsible only for CC policymaking. The director of the CC was solely responsible for a second-level review of all protocols approved by an ICRS. These changes began in 1975 and required two full years to implement. DHEW regulations specified that "community interests" should be represented by IRB members with nonscience backgrounds. Clergy, lawyers, public administrators, and teachers of ethics were added to the CC review groups. John Fletcher was invited by the clinical director of the NCI to join its ICRS in 1975.

In 1976, Mortimer Lipsett became director of the CC. In his first year, he faced review of at least 200 new protocols and annual review of hundreds more. He recognized a need for ethical consultation and for a current review of the many ethical issues that arise in clinical investigation. In discussions with the medical board about employing a bioethicist, Lipsett was strongly supported by Sheldon Wolff, clinical director of the National Institute of Allergy and Infectious Diseases (NIAID), who had assisted Fletcher in a study of consent practice in 1966–68. Ross, who had become deputy director of the CC, also favored the idea of another source of impartial and direct help in research ethics. His own study had revealed many inconsistencies in review practices. Following an interview, Lipsett offered the job to Fletcher.

Prior to employment of a bioethicist, the NIH's external and internal programs had been carefully scrutinized to increase protection of subjects' rights and safety. NIH's leaders knew that serious problems existed in both programs. An entire commission and a strengthened administrative arm were needed to improve the extramural standards. The need for a specialist in research ethics at the CC was not controversial in 1977, but it was not clear what an internal bioethicist ought to do. Several years of interaction between NIH officials and "ethicists" preceded, but did not heavily influence, the decision to employ one. Ethicists wrote papers and testified for the national commission. They also occasionally attended NIH conferences, leaving variable impressions of their value.

The decision to hire Fletcher as bioethicist was based on three factors: (1) Lipsett's needs arising from research review and his interest in educating clinical investigators, (2) the readiness of veteran researchers like Wolff and Ross to work with a bioethicist, sparked by their commitment to high standards for patient care, and (3) Fletcher's availability and familiarity with the CC.

How Did the Role Evolve?

As a discipline, bioethics in the United States was practiced mainly in teaching, research, and writing about value conflicts that consistently arise in the relationship of science to the larger society. The appearance of bioethicists on official governmental panels to help study ethical issues probably began with Albert Jonsen's role on the National Heart, Lung, and Blood Institute's (NHLBI's) Artificial Heart Assessment Panel in 1972–73.[29] Jonsen was also probably the first practicing ethics consultant in a major medical center (the University of California at San Francisco). He was employed in 1973 with a directive to "be a consultant" (personal communication, 1982). In

the late 1970s, some medical institutions employed philosophers or theologians to teach ethics and other courses in the
humanities. Some new, clinical approaches to teaching
bioethics also emerged. Harvard's School of Medicine introduced "ethics rounds" conducted by a physician, a philosopher,
and a historian of medicine.[30] Today, medical centers regularly
invite ethicists or physicians trained in ethics to participate in
rounds or case conferences when patient care decisions are
made or reviewed.[31,32] Philosophers teach and assist with the
preparation of medical students.[33] The CC may have been the
first research center in the United States to employ a bioethicist
to assist in day-to-day moral problems in clinical investigation.
Today, however, many academic medical centers and private
research facilities employ or consult with bioethicists.

Fletcher foresaw that the practical requirements of the
work would need the director's help, especially since a large
body of rules and regulations governing clinical research
already existed. Since the assignment called for direct involvement with medical staff and patients, and the role of a bioethicist in a clinical research unit was still unshaped, the
bioethicist's office was established in the office of the director,
to lend weight to the new position and to make it possible for
the bioethicist to call for the director's support when the need
arose.

EARLY ACTIVITIES AND REQUESTS FOR HELP

Lipsett first assigned Fletcher to assist him in second-level
research review and to educate CC staff about bioethical issues
in research. Lipsett's strategy for the role of bioethicist was to
emphasize the educational task. Lipsett's 20 years of experience
as a clinical investigator in the NCI, and as branch chief in
endocrinological studies in the NICHHD, were at Fletcher's
disposal to help him learn the ways and preferences of biomedical researchers. Lipsett advised Fletcher to keep a visible
but nonthreatening profile. He wanted bioethics to become an
acceptable source of help to those who were interested in it for
their own needs.

In the first months, Fletcher engaged in several activities to meet with others and educate. He (1) interviewed each clinical director and several senior investigators about their needs and expectations for a bioethics program; (2) led seminars by invitation for nurses, physicians, and social workers; (3) attended medical rounds, by invitation, in several institutes; (4) attended weekly interdisciplinary case conferences in the surgery branch of the NCI; (5) participated weekly for six months in a meeting with patients and staff of the schizophrenia studies program of the National Institute of Mental Health (NIMH), centered on the patients' understanding, doubts, and fantasies about the research and informed consent;[34] (6) introduced department heads, nurses, and other staff to the concerns of bioethics in clinical research; and (7) provided a training session for outside members of the ICRSs and encouraged them to alert him to problems.

Six requests for consultation about bioethical problems were made in the first three months. The problems involved patient consent or conflicts between the needs of patient care and the needs of research. No previous structure or experience existed in the CC to deal with specific requests for ethics consultations. Since everyone involved was dealing with a new situation, communication problems emerged in the earliest requests for help.

The entry of a bioethicist into the clinical research unit, even though he had been invited by a staff member, evoked diverse responses. Early talks and interviews with clinical directors revealed that the bioethicist was widely viewed as (1) a policeman, (2) a spy for the director, (3) an adversary or obstacle to research, (4) a teacher, and (5) a consultant. His involvement was viewed by most as a danger to researchers' interests.

When help was requested from the bioethicist, some physicians felt a loss of control or implicit judgment on their ability to manage a case. The reaction was evident even when the requester was the attending physician, but it was more severe when the request arose from a colleague, nurse, or social worker. Disputes between the disciplines typically accompanied ethical questions about the best interests of a research subject who was also very ill. The history of personal and professional relationships between "colleagues" also converged on ethical problems. Each institute was perceived by leaders as a separate "territory." In addition, polarization increased in quarters still concerned about the elevation of the director of the CC to a much stronger role in practical ethics.

Friction, suspicion, and hostility characterized the relationship between the bioethicist and some key staff members in these shaky consultations. Lipsett often discussed these matters with Fletcher and acknowledged the difficulties inherent in forging a role in a setting where sensitivities about physicians' ethical character are so deeply etched by training and tradition.

PSYCHIATRIC CONSULTATION

Many snags and role conflicts emerged in the first year of work. Fletcher was frequently embroiled in older disputes that had little bearing on the case at hand. His role seemed to be resented or regarded with suspicion in the parts of the CC where he most wanted to be effective. When a consultation provoked hostility, opposition, or blame from physicians, the emotional dynamics often superseded the case's ethical problem. The difficult family dynamics of some of the cases complicated the consideration of the ethical alternatives. Realizing that he was at a standoff in his first year of work, Fletcher asked for the help of a psychiatric consultant. Clinical center administration contracted with Maxwell Boverman for his services as psychiatric consultant to the bioethicist.

Boverman and Fletcher met frequently in the context of the bioethicist's work. He joined Fletcher to interview 35 patients and family members about their experience in the consent process.[35] They made walk-rounds to meet staff nurses, physicians, and other key figures. They also met weekly for a two-hour review of cases and problems. They interviewed Lipsett, Ross, other key administrators, head nurses, social workers, and several clinical directors about the role of the bioethicist and issues in communication. These interviews gave valuable feedback about the bioethicist's performance and contributed toward Lipsett's goal of improved communication.

Ross then convened a small communication group which met weekly for two years to address problems in communication. Members presented cases and attempted to help one another learn to be less defensive and not to back away from conflict. Boverman acted as consultant to the group. Membership shifted (with the exception of Ross, Fletcher, and Boverman), and several administrators and a physician participated in the group. Their strengthened communication reinforced other efforts by CC administrators to clarify lines of responsibility between the office of the director and the work of the institutes.

As psychiatric consultant, Boverman was directly involved in some subsequent cases:

1. The aggrieved husband of a patient was referred to Ross's office with a complaint that "no informed consent was taking place" between the couple and the physician because of personality problems and disagreements. The husband had already made copious notes and threatened to contact outsiders and newspapers unless the situation was resolved. Ross referred the husband to the bioethicist, who involved the psychiatric consultant, with the husband's agreement. Ross helped to convene meetings to discuss the complaint with the physicians involved in the case. The problem was resolved by a series of meetings between patient, family, and physicians in which differences were directly aired and consent obtained daily for each new step in the management of the case.

2. A physician inadvertently admitted a 21-year-old man, a Jehovah's Witness, to a protocol that randomized him to major surgery. The physician, realizing his error, called the bioethicist for help. The bioethicist involved the psychiatrist in a large meeting with fam-

ily, church members, and physicians to discuss the
ethical issue of refusing blood transfusions after surgery. The physician explained the high risk of death.
The patient refused whole blood but agreed to proceed
with artificial blood products. Everyone agreed that
the patient had the right to refuse based on religious
principles. The patient was discharged feeling that the
CC had respected his religious freedom, and he died
one year later.

3. A 24-year-old man with a diagnosis of schizophrenia
was referred by his psychiatrist to participate in a
double-blind, crossover study of the therapeutic benefits of hemodialysis. The patient's parents objected to
his participation, pointing to the risks to him and them
of therapeutic failure. Staff were eager to recruit him.
The parents threatened to sue if they proceeded with
the study. The issue was the right of the patient to
proceed without the agreement of his parents. The
bioethicist was asked for help with the dispute and
involved the psychiatrist in a meeting with the staff
and patient. The staff eventually decided not to enter
the patient in the protocol because of the parents'
strong opposition.[36]

Following these jointly conducted consultations, the psychiatrist had more data on which to base a constructive
approach to role conflicts. He also helped the bioethicist with
insights into the "triangulation" process; that is, when two parties isolate another as the source of the problem.

In addition to more active collaboration with the bioethicist, the psychiatric consultant was asked by the chief of nursing services to meet with nurses in a new intensive care unit of
the CC. The stated problems were poor morale and communication problems between nurses and physicians.

The psychiatrist also learned through actual case experience. He provided valuable services, including (1) support in
an environment that was, at times, hostile; (2) help in distin-
guishing the ethical issues in a case from the emotional, legal,

administrative, and medical dimensions; (3) encouragement to stay with the ethical problem at hand and not be diverted by emotional dynamics; (4) help to remain "in circulation" even when faced with opposition or indifference; (5) help in not backing down from a position, especially if institutional rules and policies were implicated; (6) help on allied communication issues in the context of cases; and, perhaps most importantly, (7) help in shaping a supportive arrangement between the bioethicist and the CC director. Since a bioethicist has no authority to require staff to adhere to institutional rules and policies, the authority of the director had to be used in timely and effective ways.

Through these consultations, Lipsett and Fletcher more clearly discerned the limits of the bioethicist's role and determined when the director should be called on to articulate policy or intervene. The most painful role conflicts occurred when Fletcher attempted to exert authority with physicians about concrete decisions in the consent process, without calling on the director to assume this task. In the early evolution of the role, when a problem was brought to the bioethicist's attention, he sometimes found areas in which a physician's action or inaction might be questionable. At first, he took it upon himself to press these points. However, a bioethicist has no institutional authority (nor should he or she have) to order a change in the behavior of clinical investigators. The role is limited to responding to requests, gathering information, clarifying issues, and making a recommendation to the interested person and the proper authorities. Through experience, and with the help of the consultant, he learned to call on the director for support and action when the situation required it. In each new case, the director provided the needed help. In one especially hard consent situation, Lipsett personally appeared in the first part of a meeting between physicians and family members, to show to the participants how important the issue was to him and the institution, and to assure the bioethicist that the consent process was faithfully carried out. The hard feelings that had developed between the bioethicist and one of the physicians were later aired by both in the presence of the director.

In the vast majority of ethical disputes, the director and the bioethicist agreed on the final outcome. In some, however, disagreement remained, and the director acted on his own best judgment after clarifying his reasons. In only one case the bioethicist felt so strongly about a principle that he stated that he would resign rather than follow the alternative under consideration. New information and the help of others broke the impasse.

CHANGING PERCEPTIONS OF THE BIOETHICIST'S ROLE

As the bioethicist accepted the consultant's help and the director's guidance, constructive change began. He developed more effective methods in ethics consultations. When ethical issues arose, he communicated more clearly and frequently with senior supervisors and those who reported the problem. He became more skilled at identifying the ethical aspect of a problem and the parts that should be referred to others. He actively sought help from others to protect "whistle blowers." Every effort was made to create an open climate.

As the bioethicist became more familiar with the clinical situation, he was perceived as more "clinically astute," according to an interview with the clinical director. Lipsett furthered the positive change and was especially eager to dispel the perception that the bioethicist was a "spy for the director." In early 1979, he shortened the title of the position from Assistant for Bioethics to the Director to Assistant for Bioethics, in order to signify that the bioethicist worked for all clinical investigators. The position remained directly under the director, but the physical location of the office was changed, so that anyone coming for help would not feel the presence, for better or worse, of the director and other administrators.

Follow-up interviews with clinical directors in 1980–81 indicated that perceptions of the bioethicist as teacher and consultant far outweighed the more negative images of enforcer of rules (police officer), possible informant (spy), or adversary of research. The latter perception was not found at all, possibly due to Lipsett's strong efforts to expedite research review and

Fletcher's more frequent ethics consultations. The climate of hostility and danger had changed, largely due to the new strength in the support system between the director, the bioethicist, and key senior investigators. It is interesting that the communication required to resolve ethical issues became a paradigm of improved communication between persons and authorities throughout the CC.

THE FUNCTIONING ROLE OF THE BIOETHICIST

In 1977, there was little precedent for the work of an applied bioethicist in a research hospital. Some investigators in the clinical center were confused by the title itself and construed it as an indication of opposition to research. Some identified bioethics with religion, possibly because of Fletcher's clerical background. (One physician came into his office in 1977 and asked, "Where is the prayer rug?") However, subsequent interviews with clinical directors and others showed that the role evolved into three clear dimensions: teacher, consultant, and bridge to authority.

Two socioethical assumptions ultimately control the role. First, research is highly valued by modern societies as a means to act on imperatives to increase benefits to public health and to fairly extend these benefits. However, a second assumption transcends and guides the first. Research to benefit society ought not to compromise the principles of respect for persons and justice, especially by manipulation of the standard of voluntary choice to be a subject of research or by exploitation of socially vulnerable persons not in a position to make a voluntary, informed choice.

The public laws that provide the authority for NIH's programs articulate the value of biomedical research to society (Public Health Service Act, Title IV; 42 U.S.C. 281).[37] The best reflections of the national commission identify the principle of beneficence with the social benefits conferred by research. Beneficence, in the commission's Belmont Report, is understood as a primary ethical obligation with two expressions: (1) to maximize benefits, and (2) to minimize or prevent harm. The report stated that "in the case of scientific research in general, members of the larger society are obliged to recognize the longer term benefits and risks that may result from the improvement of knowledge and from the development of novel medical, psychotherapeutic, and social procedures."[38]

The second socioethical assumption posits a higher obligation than social benefits; namely, respect for the ethical grounds on which society permits individuals and groups to be involved as objects of study. Two brief examples illustrate this stronger ethical claim. First, one ought to praise another who participates in research as a subject, especially when it is truly unknown what benefit will be conferred on the subject. Much can be learned for the benefit of others, and group altruism deserves praise. But it is morally inappropriate to blame a person who refuses to participate in a nontherapeutic study or an early trial of a new and unproven therapy. Group altruism is limited by the ethics of reciprocal altruism. If one receives nothing in return for one's gift, the freedom of choice to give it is virtually absolute. Further, it is especially unfitting to blame a person who withdraws from a study after it begins, even though allocated resources are lost. One deserves blame in moral relationships with society and individuals only when proven standards of reciprocity are refused or betrayed. The most unethical act in research is to manipulate the ethics of altruism and place blame or undue pressure on an unwilling subject. The voluntary consent of the subject (or his or her representative) to research is a sine qua non. Research ethics is a subset of medical ethics. In Western medical ethics, even when a patient's rights are in conflict with a patient's welfare, as in the case of the right to refuse treatment, society has increasingly given the adult the right to make a decision. The society values self-determination highly. Accordingly, when the needs of research threaten to compromise a subject's welfare, research must give way to the ethics of medical care. The needs of the individual prevail.

The applied bioethicist in the CC must work within the tension of competing values which subordinate clinical research to the ethics of medicine. The ethics of medicine are set within general social-ethical systems that guide major institutions, their activities, and roles.

THE BIOETHICIST AS TEACHER

Formal teaching at the clinical center involves lectures and seminars on research ethics, placed within the general orientation described above. Lectures are given by invitation, with the following topics addressed: (1) the ethical principles that ought to guide researchers and review bodies, (2) paradigm cases that illustrate the need for protection of subjects and researchers, and (3) the special moral and ethical problems that confront clinical investigators. Talks are routinely given to new physicians who come to the CC for training in clinical investigation, to each new group of normal volunteers, and periodically to nursing and social work services. Following the talk, time is given for questions and evaluations of actual ethical practices in the CC. Meetings with normal volunteers are especially good opportunities to provide information about incidents that indicate a need to improve ethical practices.

Because the educational task is of primary importance, the teaching role is shared by a number of employees. An interdisciplinary committee was formed in 1979 to plan educational programs for CC staff on nonmedical aspects of patient care in a research facility. The group's task was to identify timely nonmedical issues in the CC and to translate them into effective educational events. The first program was on data confidentiality, coinciding with the inauguration of a computer-assisted system for handling patient records and information. A second program (1981), "Ethics in Clinical Research," provided a historical perspective on research ethics, two brief talks by younger researchers on their personal experience with ethical problems, and a panel made up of the members of various health care disciplines who discussed issues with the audience. Through the agenda committee, each discipline has a voice in selecting group ethical concerns.

In 1979, the bioethicist first offered a two-hour, twelve-week course, "Problems in Bioethics," in a curriculum sponsored by the Foundation for the Advancement of Education in the Sciences (FAES).[39] This course still continues, essentially in the same form. NIH continues to offer courses through the FAES to help in the continuing education of employees in the life sciences.

Two other forms of teaching are experiential and clinically oriented. The bioethicist attends weekly medical rounds in a ward for endocrine disorders and makes weekly rounds of patients with genetic disorders with members of the Inter-Institute Genetics Program. The role of the bioethicist in rounds is to raise ethical questions for discussion, clarify ethical questions in a case, and follow up when help is requested for an ethical problem with a patient. Conversely, rounds give the bioethicist a rich opportunity to hear clinical investigators discuss and debate current approaches to innovative therapy, and to generate new goals in research. Researchers regularly see the bioethicist when new ideas in research are generated at the patient's bedside. The protocols that evolve from these discussions are later ethically evaluated by the bioethicist in the context of research review. Readiness to accept practical bioethics is heavily dependent on the guidance of the leader of the institution and the expertise of the bioethicist. In the past, the two units that most readily requested and received on-the-scene ethical help were a unit started by Lipsett and a service related to Fletcher's major research interest, the ethics of applied genetic knowledge.

Training is an important aspect of NIH's mission. Between 1978 and 1987, seven bioethics interns trained under the supervision of the bioethicist. The interns, who worked alongside the bioethicist and observed his activities, included a teacher of medical ethics from a local medical school, a seminarian, a lawyer from Greece, a first-year medical student, two teachers of philosophy, and a graduate student in religious studies, who sought clinical experiences for their own educational and professional development. The occupational diversity of the interns illustrates the increasing interest in the moral problems raised by clinical research.

THE BIOETHICIST AS CONSULTANT

Two distinct activities characterize the bioethicist's consulting role: responding to requests for help with ethical issues in the context of research planning and formal review; and responding to requests from clinical investigators, nurses, and others, including patients and family members, for help with ethical problems.

Ethical Issues in Research Review

Ethical questions often arise in the planning stage of research. For example, is randomization ethically as well as scientifically indicated? Is a placebo justified? How many subjects are truly required and how will they be recruited? Will the consent process present any problems? What information will be disclosed?

Some investigators consult the bioethicist with ethical questions before committing the written protocol to final form and official review. Early consultation prepares the principal investigator (PI) for formal review and helps the protocol move through the process with fewer major changes. The bioethicist serves as an "early warning system" for ethical issues that lie ahead.

For example, in 1982, the chief of the CC's new intensive care unit (ICU) planned a broad and complex study of patients who go into septic shock after being immunosuppressed. Patients were to be admitted to the ICU from the institutes in which this condition was most likely to occur (e.g., NCI and NIAID). He recognized that a major consent issue was involved, since the patients were desperately ill and sometimes even unconscious. Department of Health and Human Services regulations prevent research procedures "of more than minimal risk" with subjects whose informed consent might be compromised, when the research is designed only to obtain knowledge and not to provide a therapeutic benefit to the subject.[40] The physician consulted the bioethicist about the consent issue and the next-of-kin proxy consent in an original design to study a cardiac function by left ventricular heart catheterization. This procedure was the only investigative feature of a study with many feasible diagnostic or therapeutic benefits. The protocol was gradually reshaped so that every procedure was clinically indicated and promised benefit to a patient in septic shock. A new plan for consent was devised so that no patient unaccompanied by a family member would be involved in the study. This helped to avoid the use of proxies who might be biased toward research or unfamiliar with the patient.

Another setting for bioethics consultation is in the ICRS itself. There are 10 to 15 members in ten review bodies. Members are scientists and physicians from various disciplines. Each ICRS also has at least two nongovernment members who are not scientists. These "lay" members are lawyers, clergymen, public administrators, teachers of ethics, and retired and elected officials.

Occasionally, an ICRS calls on the bioethicist to help resolve an unusual ethical problem. At one point, for example, the bioethicist and a senior scientist met with an ICRS whose members believed that a protocol involving significant risk was being pushed on them by officials with biased interests in its approval. After careful review, the consultants recommended changes to decrease some risks, and the ICRS approved the changes. Another ethical problem in the review system addressed by Lipsett and Fletcher was possible conflict of interest when a protocol was presented to the ICRS by a scientist who was also scientific director or clinical director of the institute. The petitioner also had influential administrative and budgetary authority over many of the subpanel's members. A new policy was designed that required such protocols to be reviewed by an ICRS of another institute (augmented by special consultants with expertise in the PI's field, if necessary).

After receiving a protocol and a consent form for review, the bioethicist prepares a memorandum for the director that recommends (1) approval, (2) approval with changes, or (3) withholding approval until questions are answered. Rarely, the protocol contains problems of risk and benefit that remain to be resolved. The consent form is the main subject of a typical memorandum. It stresses clarity of explanation, especially in risk/benefit information. It may raise questions about procedures in the study, such as selection criteria, or call the director's attention to disputes in the ICRS's minutes about particular points. The director's comments about ethical issues are usually presented in the form of questions to be answered. Occasionally, the director will instruct the PI, after consultation, to avoid a procedure.

After the 1981 regulations, consent forms composed by PIs showed steady improvement in clarity on risk/benefit information and in the use of the elements required to ensure adequate consent. Standard forms provide the routine sections of the consent. The investigator has only to draft a text that discloses risks, benefits, purpose, description of procedures, and therapeutic alternatives. Each research subject is given a copy of the protocol's consent form to keep. Many PIs give the form to the patient to read with a family member or friend, prior to a meeting to discuss the issues. This technique has proven effective in improving the patient's understanding.[41]

Ethical Problems in a Clinical Research Hospital

A few selected cases are presented here to show the range of ethical dilemmas in a research hospital.

1. A liaison psychiatrist asked the bioethicist for a consultation about an informed consent problem with a 31-year-old homosexual male admitted for study of multiple infections and collapse of immunological functions. (This case occurred before the designation of AIDS to this disease.) The patient's parents had been alienated from him for years and did not accompany him to the CC. The psychiatrist believed the patient might have organic brain disease. The bioethicist and the psychiatrist saw the patient with the attending physician. Some improvement in mental status had occurred since the psychiatrist's previous visit. The bioethicist recommended that the patient be asked to consent to the tests but that his parents be

called immediately and told of the tests and the seriousness of the prognosis. The psychiatrist telephoned the parents, who came on the same day and remained until the patient died six weeks later.

2. A surgeon was invited by the bioethicist to meet following an interdisciplinary case conference in which the surgeon was criticized by staff nurses and others about an issue of informed consent. A 14-year-old boy faced amputation of a leg for sarcoma. His overly protective parents refused to allow the boy to see and meet with another child who had already had a leg amputated. There was a need for chest biopsy to determine the presence of further metastases. The biopsy was to be carried out during primary surgery for sarcoma. The issue was whether to tell the boy about the biopsy. The surgeon, upon the urging of the parents, decided that the boy was too "fragile" to learn of the additional procedure. He withheld the information from the patient, who woke up after surgery and asked why his chest hurt. Nurses were angry that they were confronted by a patient who, in their view, should have been previously informed. After discussing the situation with the psychiatric consultant, the bioethicist listened to the surgeon's reflections on the conflict. The surgeon asked whether a responsibility still existed to the patient. The bioethicist recommended that the boy be told about the nondisclosure and the surgeon's conflict, in the presence of the parents. The recommendation was carried out by the surgeon.

3. Physicians were concerned about possible psychological damage if they disclosed the fact of an XY karyotype to a 25-year-old woman with gonadal dysgenesis who had been successfully treated with experimental hormone therapy. The issue was discussed in rounds. The bioethicist and the patient's physician conferred about a strategy of disclosure. On the bioethicist's recommendation, the physician asked the patient if she

would be interested in learning more about the origin of the disorder. She assured him that she was interested. He explained the "chromosomal accident" and cautioned her that she might hear less informed persons refer to her as having a "male" biological identity. She said that she understood, since she had been a genetics major in college (a fact that her physician had not known). She thanked him for his clear explanation and showed no signs later of emotional distress.

4. A psychologist reported to the bioethicist that he was concerned about the resistance of a four-year-old female to a research procedure essential to a therapeutic study of childhood growth problems. The parent wanted the child to receive therapy. The psychologist was concerned that the child might be permanently harmed if she were forced to undergo the procedure. The psychologist had written the child's physician a memorandum but had received no reply. The bioethicist contacted the child's physician and arranged a meeting between the two professionals and their supervisors. The bioethicist chaired the meeting. Following a full discussion, a strategy was outlined for a psychiatric consultation to recommend whether the child should continue in the study. A child psychiatrist spent time with the child and her parents. Play therapy was recommended to determine the child's feelings about the procedure. The child became more cooperative. Follow-up revealed that she had accepted the test without any coercion and that the psychologist was satisfied with the outcome. Follow-up after six months found the mother to be relieved and grateful for everyone's interest in her child.

Requests for ethics consultation about problems with patients or volunteers increased from 12 in 1978 to 55 in 1983. Over 90 percent of requests originated from staff physicians or nurses. Ethical questions are seldom raised about investigators who might have violated research ethics by manipulating the weakened autonomy of very ill or vulnerable subjects. In the first six years of the bioethics program, the bioethicist was consulted about this problem on only three occasions. In only one case was there information to support the allegation. A more common and complex compromise of research ethics stems from a rarely examined tendency in the institution to subtly exploit the special vulnerability of those investigators, patients, and normal volunteers who believe themselves to be in the "best medical research center in the world." A whole institution, generations of physicians, and sick and healthy persons labor together to make the NIH's work possible. Special help is needed, however, to separate illusion from hope and fact from fantasy. Bioethics, like any practice of self-examination, must not stop with individuals. The institution and its structures require analysis.

The ethics consultant and his or her colleagues are involved in a widening circle of cooperative and conflicting altruistic endeavors.[42] For example, the willingness of desperately sick persons to benefit others coincides with the willingness of scientists to suspend their favorite scientific convictions and conduct clinical trials in the search for less biased findings. On the other hand, the goals of science sometimes conflict with the best interests of hopelessly ill persons who serve in experiments. Physician-investigators who submit to their own passion for seeking answers can exploit patients who submit to their own desire to make their suffering make a difference.

One of the most dangerous and, fortunately, rarest events in research involves the betrayal of the researcher by the subject. The consequences may be tragic when a patient or normal volunteer successfully deceives the conscientious but unwary investigator about vital information relevant to the capacity to be a subject.[43]

Methods for Ethics Consultations

The bioethicist must develop rational methods for ethics consultation. The first step is to decide if the problem is truly an ethical one. Should it be referred to someone else? Enough information must be collected to answer that question. Callers often have conflicting views about what constitutes an "ethical" dilemma. In addition, the ethicist must determine whether there is real or potential danger to the welfare of a patient or normal volunteer or to those who carry out research. Clinical investigators often forget that research ethics exist to protect them from censure, discipline, or even "debarment," because a moral error which might reasonably have been prevented causes harm to persons for whom they are responsible. Problems are sometimes determined to be purely legal, administrative, or religious, and further referral must be made. If an ethical problem exists, the consultation begins.

The second step is to ascertain what kind of help the requester needs. Most often, he or she wants a recommendation as to a proper course of action when one or more choices are in conflict. At other times, the caller wants to talk "off the record" about the concern. Requests for confidentiality present problems, because the bioethicist can become entrapped in pledges that constitute breaches of institutional rules or law. The consultant may then find it difficult to mobilize the appropriate resources to solve the problem. The bioethicist should ask the caller to restrain the need for confidentiality until enough is known about the problem to proceed. The caller is asked to trust the bioethicist and to describe the problem without implicating others by name.

The third step is to establish the facts of the case. Often, the principal actors in a case must be interviewed separately or together. If the problem involves a patient or a normal volunteer, the person must be interviewed by the bioethicist, so that statements about the patient's condition, competence, or state of grievance are compared with the patient's experience.

The fourth step is to make a verbal or written recommendation about alternatives, if it is requested. When recommending a course of action, the bioethicist knows that the requester may disagree. When the recommended course of action involves institutional rules, and there is disagreement about the relevance of those rules, there can be further trouble. The bioethicist is a teacher, not an enforcer, of rules. Simply rehearsing the relevant rules usually suffices to provoke compliance.

When the bioethicist and a senior physician disagree about a proper course of action in a particular case, the bioethicist must withdraw after giving a recommendation and informing the physician's superior about the disagreement. One major difference between an ethics consultation and a medical consultation is that it is more difficult for the bioethicist to withdraw after becoming committed to a course of action. This problem is unusual for the typical medical consultant. It is difficult to be impartial about one's own moral advice, even though impartiality has played a crucial role in the formation of a recommendation. The best remedy after a stormy, disputatious case is to talk it through with the key persons involved, encouraging learning and discouraging self-righteousness. Spite must be avoided if at all possible, since it lays the traps for future disputes. Old moral anger contaminates new conflicts, and they become even more inflamed.

Disciplinary Issues

The bioethicist may be consulted by senior officials on questions concerning the professional ethics of clinical investigators who might have violated institutional policies or procedures for review. As the inquiry into questionable conduct proceeds, the bioethicist may, if requested to do so, prepare a memorandum for the record about the ethical issue. The bioethicist does not take part in any decisions to discipline physicians or any other staff.

THE BIOETHICIST AS BRIDGE TO AUTHORITY

The bioethicist does not have the administrative authority to order anyone to work in compliance with the norms of research ethics or medical ethics. However, he or she can advise another as to the rules and the consequences of avoidance or violation. When the issue is compliance, the bioethicist must turn to higher authorities in the institutes and the CC for enforcement.

If the problem is a breach of the rules, it can be quickly referred to administrators. If, in the course of an ethics consultation, the parties become embroiled in a dispute about the applicability of rules, other authorities must resolve the issue.

Because the bioethicist's role as a bridge to authority is to help protect human subjects and investigators from the consequences of misjudgment in research, it is crucial that a nonthreatening climate prevail around the position. Those who inform the bioethicist about problems must be reassured that no punishment will follow due to the report. Supervisors can help to create a nonthreatening climate by assuring the informant that he or she did the right thing by consulting the bioethicist.

Finally, the bioethicist serves those in authority who make scientific policy and regulations to protect the human subjects of research. For example, he or she assists with discussions of long-range consequences of genetic engineering, in vitro fertilization, fetal research, and other volatile subjects in research. Further, the bioethicist drafts discussion papers for problems that will face researchers in the future. For example, when an effective test to detect presymptomatic Huntington's disease is available, what is the best way to approach screening before there is an effective therapy?

SUMMARY IN EVOLUTIONARY PERSPECTIVE

This chapter has traced the evolution of a new role in applied bioethics in the setting of clinical research. Although it has some of the same "helping" elements as the roles of chaplain, social worker, and administrator, the role is distinctive because it relies on a specialized knowledge of the ethical principles and moral conduct expected in clinical investigation. The applied or practical bioethicist is a teacher of principles and rules that ought to guide researchers. Because difficult moral choices are the occasions for requests for help, the bioethicist must be an effective consultant. Better results may be achieved when the bioethicist works in widespread, cooperative relationships with other professionals, drawing on reliable scientific or medical information related to the problem at hand. Further, psychiatric collaboration is sometimes indispensable in bioethical consultations, especially those that involve disputes among family members. Psychiatrists are also needed to examine whether harm can result from disclosure of risk or poor prognosis. Finally, the bioethicist is a link between authorities with legitimate power to resolve problems and those who bring problems to light.

The development of the role of the bioethicist at the CC of the NIH has offered a level of protection for research subjects and investigators beyond relying on the conscience of the individual physician-investigator (often invoked as the only reliable bulwark by early critics of human experimentation).[44] The practice of prior group review, which has been adopted in many nations in addition to the United States,[45] has also reduced risks to subjects. It answers with impartiality the first and foremost moral question in research: What is ethically fitting to ask of research subjects in their own interest? For society's interests? Further, what is the optimal form for assessment of risk and benefit? When provided with enough time, leadership, and institutional support, review groups develop skill and confidence in their tasks.[46,47]

Finally, the evolution of informed consent as a requirement in almost every context of biomedical research has also increased protection for human subjects. DHHS guidelines require that the consent form be given to the subject to keep, so the subject may consult with others, including family members, away from the presence and possible pressure of the interested investigator. Investigators who denounce the written form should reexamine the value of its impartiality. The investigator will have difficulty in justifying his or her contempt for "legalities" while awaiting a lawsuit brought by the subject of a painful procedure that had not been explained on the consent form. Many researchers have studied the problems of informed consent, the shortcomings of subjects' recall, and methods to improve the outcomes of the consent encounter.[48] A pilot study of involvement of family members in the consent process of the CC showed clear benefits to patient, family, and physician.[49]

Careful examination of data to show whether informed consent can be harmful or hazardous, as is often claimed, shows that this moral and legal requirement is in fact helpful to patients' mental health.[50]

As the body of knowledge concerning research ethics became larger and more specialized, the opportunity arose to provide an on-the-scene ethicist in the CC. The role provides a sounding board for ideas, issues, and implications in debates about directions in clinical research. When the rules of research ethics are in question in an actual case, the bioethicist can be a catalyst in helping clinical investigators and their associates to resolve dilemmas. The bioethicist is regarded as an ombudsman for patient interests who can also protect the mission of the institution and researchers from the harm of misjudgments.

An applied bioethicist is a useful addition to the complex and evolving system designed to protect human subjects. However, the key to the effectiveness of the role is the strong support of medical authorities in a clinical research setting. Applied bioethics is a partnership between leaders of an institution and teachers of research ethics who must become involved in the daily work of clinical research in order to be effective.

NOTES

1. The NIH includes the National Cancer Institute (NCI), the National Heart, Lung, and Blood Institute (NHLBI), the National Institute of Allergy and Infectious Diseases (NIAID), the National Institute of Arthritis, Diabetes and Digestive and Kidney Disease (NIADDKD), the National Institute of Child Health and Human Development (NICHHD), the National Institute of Aging (NIA), the National Institute of Dental Research (NIDR), the National Institute of Neurological and Communicative Diseases and Stroke (NINCDS), the National Eye Institute (NEI), and the National Institute of Mental Health (NIMH).

2. *Bonner* v. *Moran*, 126 F.2d 121 (D.C. Cir. 1941) is discussed in Jay Katz, *Experimentation with Human Beings* (New York: Russell Sage Foundation, 1972).

3. U.S. Adjutant General's Department, "The Medical Case," in *Trials of War Criminals Before Nuremberg Military Tribunals Under Control Council Law No. 10* (Washington, DC: U.S. Government Printing Office, 1947).

4. The Nuremberg Code, composed of ten principles, was drafted with the help of Dr. Andrew C. Ivy, medical consultant to the war crimes tribunal, and Dr. Leo Alexander. See Leo Alexander, "Medical Science under Dictatorship," *New England Journal of Medicine* 241 (1949): 39-47; and Jay Katz, *Experimentation with Human Beings* (New York: Russell Sage Foundation, 1972).

5. Irving Ladimer, "Human Experimentation: Medicolegal Aspects," *New England Journal of Medicine* 257 (1957): 18-24.

6. Chauncey Leake, ed., *Percival's Medical Ethics* (Baltimore: Williams and Wilkins, 1927).

7. U.S. National Institutes of Health, "Group Consideration of Clinical Research Procedures Deviating from Accepted Medical Practice or Involving Unusual Hazard," memorandum approved by Director, NIH, 1953.

8. Stuart M. Sessoms, "What Hospitals Should Know about Investigational Drugs—Guiding Principles in Medical Research Involving Humans," *Hospitals* 32 (1958): 44-64.

9. U.S. National Institutes of Health, "Participation by NIH Employees as Normal Controls in Clinical Research Projects," memorandum from NIH Director, 1954.

10. Louis G. Welt, "Reflections on the Problems of Human Experimentation," *Connecticut Medicine* 25 (1961): 75-78.

11. William Curran, "Subject Consent Requirements in Clinical Research: The Approach of Two Agencies," *Daedalus* 98 (1960): 545.

12. John C. Fletcher, "The Evolution of the Ethics of Informed Consent," in *Research Ethics*, ed. Kåre Berg and Knut E. Tranøy (New York: Alan R. Liss, 1983), pp. 187-228.

13. Elinor Langer, "Human Experimentation: New York Affirms Patients' Rights," *Science* 151 (1966): 663-65.

14. Henry K. Beecher, "Ethics and Clinical Research," *New England Journal of Medicine* 274 (1966): 1354.

15. Stephen Goldby, "Experiments at the Willowbrook State School," *Lancet* 1 (1971): 749.

16. Jane Heller, "Tuskegee Syphilis Study Revealed," *Washington Star*, July 25, 1972, p. A1.

17. James H. Jones, *Bad Blood: The Tuskegee Syphilis Experiment* (New York: Free Press, 1981).

18. Victor Cohn, "NIH Vows Not to Fund Fetus Work," *Washington Post*, April 13, 1973, p. A1.

19. U.S. Adjutant General's Department, "The Medical Case."

20. Renee C. Fox, "Advanced Medical Technology: Social and Ethical Implications," in *Essays in Medical Sociology*, ed. Renee C. Fox (New York: John Wiley, 1979), 413–61.

21. John C. Fletcher, "Realities of Patient Consent to Medical Research," *Hastings Center Studies* 1 (1973): 39–49.

22. U.S. Surgeon General, Public Health Service, "Investigations Involving Human Subjects, Including Clinical Research: Requirements for Review to Insure the Rights and Welfare of Individuals." Public policy order 129, Revised policy, July 1, 1966.

23. John C. Fletcher, "A Study of the Ethics of Medical Research" (Doctoral Dissertation, Union Theological Seminary, 1969).

24. Van Rensselaer Potter, *Bioethics: Bridge to the Future* (Englewood Cliffs, NJ: Prentice-Hall, 1971).

25. K. Danner Clouser, "Bioethics," in *Encyclopedia of Bioethics*, edited by Warren T. Reich (New York: Free Press, 1978), 115–27.

26. Robert Q. Marston, "Medical Science, the Clinical Trial, and Society," U.S. National Institutes of Health, 1972.

27. U.S. Department of Health, Education, and Welfare, "Protection of Human Subjects," General Administration, Part 46, *Federal Register* 39 (1974): 18911–20.

28. Mortimer B. Lipsett, John C. Fletcher, and Marian Secundy, "Research Reviews at NIH," *Hastings Center Report* 9 (1979): 18–21.

29. U.S. National Institutes of Health, National Heart and Lung Institute, *The Totally Implantable Artificial Heart*, DHEW Publication No. (NIH) 74-191 (Washington, DC: U.S. Government Printing Office, 1973).

30. Stanley J. Reiser, "Humanism and Fact-Finding in Medicine," *New England Journal of Medicine* 299 (1978): 950–53.

31. Mark Siegler, "A Legacy of Osler: Teaching Ethics at the Bedside," *Journal of the American Medical Association* 239 (1978): 951–56.

32. K. Danner Clouser, *Teaching Bioethics: Strategies, Problems, and Resources* (Hastings-on-Hudson, NY: The Hastings Center, 1980).

33. William Ruddick, Alan Fleischman, Mark Siegler, and Benjamin Freedman, "Philosophers in Medicine," *Hastings Center Report* 11 (April 1981): 12–22.

34. William T. Carpenter, Jr. "A New Setting for Informed Consent," *Lancet* 1 (1974): 500–501.
35. John C. Fletcher and Maxwell Boverman, "Involving the Patient's Family in Informed Consent," delivered at 88th Annual Meeting of the American Psychological Association, Montreal, Canada, 1980.
36. S. Charles Schulz, Daniel P. Van Kammen, and John C. Fletcher, "Dialysis for Schizophrenia: Consent and Costs," *Hastings Center Report* 9 (1979): 10–12.
37. John F. Sherman, "The Organization and Structure of the National Institutes of Health," *New England Journal of Medicine* 297 (1977): 18–26.
38. U.S. National Commission for the Protection of Human Subjects of Biomedical and Behavioral Research, *The Belmont Report: Ethical Principles for the Protection of Human Subjects of Research,* DHEW Publication No. (OS) 78-0012 (Washington, DC: U.S. Government Printing Office, 1978).
39. Registration for this class is limited to 12 students. Enrollment was full until 1982, when budget cuts reduced support for continuing education. An enrollment of only six resulted in cancellation. Enrollees have been physicians, nurses, technicians, and non-NIH scientists. In 1981, French W. Anderson cotaught the course with the bioethicist. The course materials feature moral and ethical reflections on problems in applied human genetics and medical care of the terminally ill.
40. U.S. Department of Health and Human Services, "Protection of Human Subjects," *Federal Register* 46 (1981): 8386.
41. Gary Morrow, Jon Gootnick, and Arthur Schmale, "A Simple Technique for Increasing Cancer Patients' Knowledge of Informed Consent to Treatment," *Cancer* 42 (1978): 793–99.
42. Peter Singer, *The Expanding Circle: Ethics and Sociobiology* (New York: Farrar, Straus, and Giroux, 1981).
43. Gina B. Kolata, "The Death of a Research Subject," *Hastings Center Report* 10 (1980): 5–6.
44. Beecher, "Ethics and Clinical Research."
45. William J. Curran, "Subject Consent Requirements in Clinical Research: An International Perspective for Industrial and Developing Countries." Unpublished, 1981.
46. Bradford H. Gray, Robert A. Cooke, and Arnold S. Tannenbaum, "Research Involving Human Subjects," *Science* 201 (1978): 1094–1101.
47. Benjamin S. Duval, Jr., "The Human Subjects Protection Commit-

tee: An Experiment in Decentralized Federal Regulation," *American Bar Association Research Journal* 1979 (1979): 573–677.

48. Alan Meisel and Loren Roth, "What We Do and Do Not Know about Informed Consent," *Journal of the American Medical Association* 246 (1981): 2473–77.
49. Fletcher and Boverman, "Involving the Patient's Family in Informed Consent."
50. Maxwell Boverman, "Mental Health Aspects of the Informed Consent Process," in *Research Ethics*, ed. Kåre Berg and Knut E. Trangøy (New York: Alan R. Liss, 1983), pp. 229–41.

5

A Comment on the Concept of Consultation

Ruth B. Purtilo

The notion that the ethicist has an appropriate service function in the health care setting is not limited to discourse among persons already engaged in such activities. The medical literature continues to promulgate the position that hospitals should employ such persons. For instance, when the *Canadian Medical Association Journal* reported that a large hospital in Montreal appointed a professional ethicist to its staff, the reason cited was that the hospital administration saw the role of the clinical ethicist as adding strength to the hospital's ability to provide good care to patients. The journal's editorial noted that "families too must be relieved to know that our staff has the kind of expertise a professional ethicist can provide on hand. It is one way we can deal with the complexity of medicine."[1] The ethicist is viewed as a vital component of good patient care and competent approaches to ethical problems facing physicians, administrators, and others.

According to standard dictionary definitions, a "consultant" is a person who provides professional advice or services regarding matters in the field of his or her special knowledge or training. In ethics, a consultation can be defined as follows:

> An *ethics consultation* can be said to occur when physicians or other members of the health care or research team recognize that they have an ethical problem or dilemma and ask a designated person to "help" with the problem. The problem usually concerns a choice to be made about the welfare of a patient or research subject but need not be restricted simply to patients. By this definition, we

mean an activity beyond attending rounds and raising ethical issues in rounds. If you attend rounds only but are not designated as an ethics consultant "on call" by request from staff, you would not yet qualify. . . .[2]

In spite of the many ways in which the activities of ethicists in hospital settings can, and increasingly do, include activities that generally fit these descriptions, the appropriateness of the "consultant" designation has not yet been determined.

CLINICAL CONSULTATION AS A MODEL

The traditional activities of a clinical consultant in the health care setting provide the most useful analogy for thinking about the ethics consultant in hospitals. In a clinical consultation, one of three scenarios results (see Figure 5.1):

1. The primary physician (i.e., physician primarily responsible for the clinical management of a patient) and patient constitute the physician-patient relationship, the unit of interaction into which a clinical consultation may be called. (Of course, there may be more than one physician or other specialist and more than one consultant.) Following a consultation, the physician will use the information provided by the consultant but may continue to be the primary person responsible for the management of the patient; the consultant's work is completed and he or she withdraws.

2. In some instances, following the consultant's visit and a subsequent evaluation of the patient's situation, the consultant is the appropriate person to resume charge of the patient's diagnostic or treatment regime. The primary physician refers the patient to the consultant's supervision.

3. The third common outcome is that, following the consultation, both the physician initially in charge and the consultant assume ongoing management of the patient's condition.

Figure 5.1
Relationships Established through Clinical Consultation

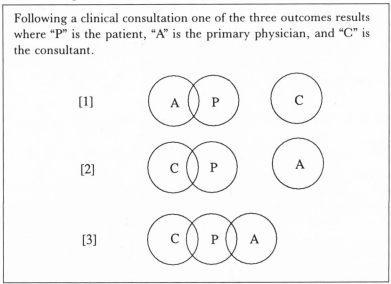

Following a clinical consultation one of the three outcomes results where "P" is the patient, "A" is the primary physician, and "C" is the consultant.

[1]   A P   C

[2]   C P   A

[3]   C P A

Given these various outcomes of clinical consultations, the limits of the analogy to the situation of the ethics consultant is evident. The only outcome of an ethics consultation is the first one. The ethicist will remain involved in the situation until the moral conflict is resolved and will become involved again if another moral conflict arises in the patient's treatment, but the relationship of primary physician and patient remains intact following the consultation. Under no circumstances would the ethics consultant become the primary caregiver in the *clinical* management of the patient. Therefore, if used too loosely, this analogy can distort perceptions of the ethicist's role.

The concept itself, however, is not necessarily incorrect. Fletcher has stated that "the more formal the consultation, the more the medical model will apply," and he has outlined important procedural aspects of consultation that are still unrefined in many consultants' activities, such as formalized mechanisms for beginning, continuing, recording, and ending a consultation.[3] Such formalization seems to highlight how fully the medical consultant model can be applied. However, it does not account for the specific demands and realities of the clinical decision-making process and the responsibilities that usually fall within the range of "clinical privileges."[4]

OTHER MODELS OF CONSULTATION

How, then, ought one to proceed? Further exploration of the consultation notion, as well as other related concepts, may prove useful. For example, Caplan's notion of "consultee-centered case consultation" is worth exploring. In consultee-centered case consultation the consultee is the physician, and the focus of the consultation is clarification regarding shortcomings in the consultee's professional functioning which are hindering an effective solution to a case at hand. The shortcomings may be (1) lack of knowledge, (2) lack of skill, (3) lack of self-confidence, or (4) lack of professional objectivity. Emphasis is placed first on improving the consultee's cognitive grasp of the situation and then on emotional mastery of the issues.

> In consultee-centered consultation, improvement in this client is a side effect, welcome though it may be, and the primary goal is to improve the consultee's capacity to function effectively in this category of case, in order to benefit many similar clients in the future. Because of this education emphasis, the consultant uses the discussion of the current case situation, not basically in order to understand the client, but in order to understand and remedy the consultee's work difficulties, as manifested in this example. . . .
>
> The significant information in this kind of consultation, therefore, comes from the consultee's subjectively determined story about the client and not from the objective reality of the client's situation. Because of this, there is usually no need for the consultant to investigate the client directly by seeing or interviewing him, and he can restrict his information to what the consultee says about the case.[5]

First, consider some strengths of such a model. Most ethicists will readily accede that much of their service work is educational, even within the context of consultation activity. This is not surprising, since most physicians and other health professionals now in practice have had little or no formal exposure to medical ethics concepts and methods during their professional preparation. In their survey of 3,000 physicians who had been out of training for five to ten years, Pellegrino and associates reported that most respondents felt they did not have adequate preparation for dealing with today's ethical problems in medicine.[6] Therefore, a concept of a consultation that has an explicitly educational focus is consistent with the expectations of many health professionals who ask for ethics "consults." Furthermore, Ackerman emphasizes the ethicist's role in clarifying values in situations of moral conflict and helping health professionals to set priorities among conflicting loyalties.[7] These examples support the idea that an ethics consultant's most important function is as an objective, expert source of information.

Second, serious consideration must be given to whether ethicists, many of whom do not hold degrees in the health professions, should have full access to medical records, patients, and other hospital resources in their attempt to gather relevant information pertaining to a case. The model of a consultee-centered consultation puts the burden of responsibility on both the health professional and the ethicist to construct a picture of the problem, thereby relieving the ethicist's worry about taking advantage of information-gathering activity usually reserved for health professionals (e.g., reading the patient's medical record in detail). Third, the model helps to focus the consultation on one case while simultaneously preparing the physician for dealing with similar cases in the future, thus enabling the clinician to draw general conclusions from the case at hand and eventually increasing the efficiency of his or her moral decision making.

The shortcomings of this model are also easy to identify. Perhaps the most troubling element is the explicit focus, not on the patient or family, but on the health professional. While we

might facilitate the process of consultation by not directly
involving the patient or others, are we also lessening the opportunity for an outcome that will benefit the patient? For example, one must consider whether the potentially harmful biases
and inconsistencies of the health professional's report will be
identified by the consultant. Caplan believes so:

> Our experience teaches us that if we listen carefully to the consul-
> tee's statements about his case, we can usually identify his biases,
> distortions, and areas of inadequate perception or planning from
> the internal consistency and inconsistency of his observations;
> from evidence of exaggeration, confusion, or stereotyping; and
> from signs of emotional overinvolvement or underinvolvement
> with one or more of the actors or situations in the client's drama.[8]

Ethicists may be less sure of themselves in this regard, particularly given their association with the health care institution
and, in many cases, their respect for or need for approval from
the health professionals who request consultation. In each case,
the patient's "side of the story" is at risk of being distorted or
blurred.

A second shortcoming of this model is that, if ethicists
adopted it in its entirety, they would convey the message that
they have all the knowledge, skills, self-confidence, and professional objectivity needed to solve all patient care problems that
are not explicitly technical and medical in nature! To mitigate
against dependence on the ethicist's general expertise, a carefully detailed explanation of the ethicist's limits and resources
would have to be communicated to potential users of the ethicist's services. Particularly critical is the need to distinguish the
ethicist's role from the psychiatrist's role, since the consultee-
centered consultation is also employed in psychiatry. Such a
distinction is needed to avoid confusion regarding the respec-
tive contributions of psychiatrists and ethicists in the resolution
of complex clinical problems. These (and probably other) considerations would have to be given arduous thought before
ethicists could affirm a wholesale adoption of the concept of
consultee-centered consultations. However, its potential as one
of several consultant models should not be neglected at this

early stage in the evolution of the consultant role in medical ethics.

A third model of consultation is that developed outside of medicine, in business, industry, engineering, law, and government relations. Emphasis in such fields is on the consultant as marketing agent, sharer of expert advice, and communications facilitator. At least one comprehensive reference book is available on the topic.[9] A New York–based organization of consultants from many different disciplines has formed a "Consultants Network," and a widely circulated *Consulting Opportunities Journal* is now available. This type of consultant model serves as a reminder to ethicists that there are several models outside of the medical context that should be considered before we decide upon a final set of criteria for our consultation activity.

Finally, the model of "consultation-liaison psychiatry" or, as it is more commonly called, "liaison psychiatry" is worth our brief consideration. The most striking feature of this model is the emphasis on communications or "bridge building" which is inherent in the concept of a liaison. The term "liaison" is from *ligure* (Latin), to bind or bring together, and also from the French *lier*, to bind or tie. According to the Oxford English Dictionary, a liaison is one who is responsible for communication among interrelated parts of an organization to insure mutual understanding, unity of action, and especially prompt and effective support from backup systems. These functions are oftened assumed by the ethicist. Lipowski, who developed the notion of liaison psychiatry, stresses the function of the liaison-psychiatrist as mediator, one who links groups, organizations, or other units, allowing effective collaboration to take place.[10] This is a common outcome of ethics consultations.

The liaison-psychiatrist is a person whose work may be prospective as well as responsive.[11] He or she may seek out potential problems and bring them to the attention of other clinicians, rather than simply waiting for requests to see a patient. If ethicists were to adopt the role of liaison, it would help to explain why they engage in prospective activities such

as identifying the need for a given policy and offering suggestions for how to avoid future problems in a ward or unit.

However, the similarities between the liaison-psychiatrist
and the ethicist are limited, and the adoption of this model may
be counterproductive for all involved. For example, if the ethicist adopts this role, again there is danger that the roles of the
psychiatrist and the ethicist will become confused. Second, the
method of liaison psychiatry is to conduct interviews with
patients, an activity that poses several serious problems for the
ethicist. Finally, there is a worry that the prospective work of a
liaison-ethicist would foster the erroneous image of the ethicist
as a moral watchdog searching the wards for perpetrators of
ethical misdemeanors and felonies.

REFLECTION

Where are we in our search for an appropriate model to guide
the service functions of ethicists in health care settings? This
excursion into the richness of the notion of consultant and
consultant-liaison should spur us to continue an exploration
into the best and most relevant interpretation for our purposes.
In the meantime, the medical literature has ample information
on the notion of effective consultations in the medical setting.
An article by Goldman, Lee, and Rudd offers "Ten Commandments for Effective Consultations," most of which could help
ethicists to understand the process of consultation as it is inter-
preted in its rather specific form in the medical setting.[12] The
social sciences literature also helps to delineate the purposes
and dynamics of consultations in the medical setting. A paper
entitled "Control in the Medical Consultation: Organizing
Talk in a Situation Where Co-Participants Have Differential
Competence" describes the ways in which interactional control
operates.[13] Anyone wishing to be an effective consultant should
take note of the author's description of the ways in which
orderly and topically relevant sequences of speech are
employed in a situation where two or more specialists come
together to solve a problem.

Finally, further exploration of the ethicist's role should

consider the following questions: Is the consultant role one that suits the activities of the ethicist in the wide variety of health care settings in which he or she may become employed? To what extent are we further individuating ourselves as important persons in the health care setting by assuming the function of and terminology of "consultant"? Are there other more appropriate means to this end? If we continue to develop the notion of consultation, where in the literature of health care disciplines and the literature of consultantship should we turn next for sound advice on how to refine the concept as it applies to us?

NOTES

1. Jane Wilson, "Editorial," *Canadian Medical Association Journal* 132 (1985): 189–90.
2. John C. Fletcher and Albert R. Jonsen, Letter to Conferees, September 28, 1982.
3. See Chapter 11.
4. See Chapter 1.
5. Gerald Caplan, *Theory and Practice of Mental Health Consultation* (New York: Basic Books, 1970), 125–26.
6. Edmund Pellegrino, et al., "Relevance and Utility of Courses in Medical Ethics: A Survey of Physicians' Perceptions," *Journal of the American Medical Association* 253 (1985): 49–53.
7. Terrence Ackerman, "Role Conflicts in Ethics Consultation," presented at the First National Conference on Ethics Consultation in Health Care, Bethesda, Maryland, October 7, 1985.
8. Caplan, *Theory and Practice of Medical Health Consultation*, 126.
9. Herman Holtz, *How to Succeed as an Independent Consultant* (New York: John Wiley and Sons, 1983).
10. Z. J. Lipowski, "Consultation-Liaison Psychiatry: An Overview," *American Journal of Psychiatry* 131 (1974): 623–30.
11. Thomas Hackett, "Beginnings: Liaison Psychiatry in a General Hospital," in *MGH Handbook of General Hospital Psychiatry*, ed. T. Hackett and E. H. Cassem (St. Louis: C. V. Mosby, 1978), 1–4.
12. Lee Goldman, Thomas Lee, and Peter Rudd, "Ten Commandments for Effective Consultations," *Archives of Internal Medicine* 143 (1983): 1753–55.

13. David Hughes, "Control in the Medical Consultation: Organizing Talk in a Situation Where Co-Participants Have Differential Competence," *Sociology* 16 (1982): 359–75.

6

Ethics Consultation with Hospital Employees in Complex Medical Settings

Anne J. Davis

Much of the literature in bioethics addresses ethical issues and problems regarding the relationship between the physician and the patient. Some of this writing seems to reflect a kind of social and clinical cocoon, whereby the doctor-patient relationship is the only important interaction. While the doctor-patient relationship is unique, both legally and ethically, the ethics in many situations are often far more complicated than this literature would have us believe.

With the advancement of science and technology and the socioeconomic factors that place the hospital at the center of medical care, a complex division of labor has developed that involves many individuals other than the physician and the patient. At the turn of this century, physicians constituted about 80 percent of all medical care deliverers, while today they account for about 12 percent of this population. Bioethics as a field has not really come to grips with this fact, but tends to operate on a model of the "good old days," where one physician rather than three or four specialists cared for the patient, and the physician was the only health care professional involved in the patient's care.

Several authors have focused on the general nature of the nurse-physician relationship.[1,2] A study concerning the perception of ethical problems by staff in acute care units of a university hospital revealed that perceived ethical problems tended to fall into these categories: (1) questions concerning how aggressively medical treatment should be pursued, including whether or not to resuscitate the patient, and (2) questions about patient preference and informal consent.[3]

While this study found little difference in the types of cases reported by nurses and physicians, it did reveal a clear difference in the perception of conflicts within the health care team. Nurses were aware of differences of opinion between nurses and physicians, but physicians were not aware of these conflicts. This situation can be explained in part by the nature of the working relationship.[4] In addition, physicians see themselves as accountable to other physicians and to patients and families, but not to nurses. Yet, the failure to address differences of opinion impedes optimum, humane care.

The fact remains that nurses spend far more time with hospitalized patients and their families than do doctors, and nurses are more apt to be aware of the patient's and the family's feelings. Nurses play a central role in patient care, and their perceptions of ethical problems may be more acute than those of physicians.

This chapter will identify and describe some of the issues that arise for the other 88 percent of care providers in complex medical settings. One of the interesting issues here is that, while most physicians who bring patients to the hospital are male (although this is changing), most of the other 88 percent of care providers are female and are employees who have a very different relationship to the institution. The dynamics of this situation surrounding the patient determine which problems are labeled as ethical by this group and how they may or may not attempt to deal with them. This chapter also raises some of the issues that the consultant faces in working with this group of professional employees.

The University of California, San Francisco, one of the nine campuses in the state university system, is a health science campus with schools of dentistry, medicine, nursing, and pharmacy. The hospitals, which consist of two acute care facilities and a psychiatric institute, all serve as clinical areas for students, interns, residents, and graduate students in nursing. In addition, numerous students in both the physical and social sciences study on campus. The inpatient hospitals' bed capacity is 560, and 800 registered nurses are employed. Like all such large health science complexes, the University of California, San Francisco has a three-part mission: clinical service, teaching, and research. Selected nurses in the hospital nursing department have unsalaried teaching appointments in the school of nursing, and some of the nursing faculty have unsalaried clinical appointments in nursing service. As an ethics consultant, I serve in one of these positions and am asked to come to the units for ethics rounds. While I sometimes receive calls from physicians or social workers, I am usually called by a nurse and, specifically, by a clinical nurse specialist.

Ethics rounds occur only when a situation has been defined as an ethical dilemma, and they do not occur on a routine basis. I am usually called to the hospital when the situation is considered urgent by the staff, although occasionally a long-term problem (one in which the staff perceive a pattern) is reported. In many of these problem situations, the attending physician is not available for discussions with the family or the staff, and this becomes a major part of the overall problem.

Since my responsibility is to the nursing department, I have no formal link to the clinical ethics committee. However, individuals in the nursing department are members of the committee, and communication channels are maintained in this manner.

Three types of ethical consultation are typical: (1) the entire staff works with a patient; (2) the nurses, residents, interns, social worker, and physical therapist work with the patient; and (3) only the nurses work with the patient. The attending physician is missing in the latter two categories, which often means that the system of communication has disintegrated between the attending physician and the others who care for the patient. When the consultation is limited to the nursing staff, it usually means that they have identified the physician as part of the problem and that the problem affects them more than it affects other staff members. Two typical cases are outlined below.

CASE STUDY I

Mr. X was terminally ill and near death, according to clinical judgments of the medical staff. He was no longer able to speak in his own best interest. The attending physician met with the two family members, both of whom were physicians themselves, and all had agreed that the patient would want treatment withdrawn given his present situation and prognosis. The attending physician went out of town and wrote no orders as a follow-up to the meeting with the family. The staff was concerned both about the doctor's failure to follow through and about the course of their own clinical behavior with this patient. While the attending physician was still away, I was asked to consult with them. Everyone else involved in the care of this patient attended the ethics consultation. After serious deliberations, it was decided that (1) there would be no resuscitation; (2) medication for the patient's respiratory infection would be discontinued; and (3) the tube feeding, which was causing a major bowel problem and in turn a serious skin breakdown, would be discontinued. The resident wrote the order discontinuing these aspects of treatment. The staff worked diligently to see that Mr. X received the best and most humane care they could possibly give. Several days later, the attending physician returned and wrote orders to reinstate the former care plan, to resuscitate, to give medication, and to tube feed. In short, all of the decisions, made on the basis of input from the family members and the outcome of the ethics consultation, were overturned.

Needless to say, the entire staff, from chief resident to nursing aide, was upset at this action. The attending physician's rationale was unclear to the staff, and when the clinical nurse specialist approached him, she did not receive an answer to her question. Based on the clinical and ethical concerns of the staff, this nurse began to take other actions to resolve what the staff continued to define as an ethical problem. She called the patient's son, a physician, and told him what had occurred. He then contacted the attending physician, who discontinued the treatment plan; the patient died shortly thereafter.

CASE STUDY II

A well-known transplant surgeon called the unit and indicated that he was bringing a potential patient, Mrs. M, to the unit. He specifically asked the nurses to move any transplant patients who were not doing well to a part of the unit where Mrs. M would not see them. The physician wanted her to see only those patients who were having a smooth postoperative course. The nurses were angry about this for two reasons: (1) they thought this request involved them in a deceitful act toward Mrs. M and that it inconvenienced the other patients; (2) they also resented the use of a scarce resource, nursing staff, to move beds around the unit. When the nursing staff approached the surgeon about their concerns on this matter, he essentially told them to tend to their nursing and he would make these sorts of decisions. The next day he brought them a box of candy. They found this action so insulting that they asked for an ethics consultation.

After an ethics round, the nurses had a meeting with the surgeon during which they outlined their concerns and the reasons for them. No similar request has been made since the discussion. In fact, there seems to be more open communication on the unit concerning ethical issues in general.

DISCUSSION

These two cases obviously have some similarities. One similarity is the lack of involvement of the attending physician in the ethics consultation. Both cases also indicate the absence of an open working relationship in which the ethical dimensions of the situations can be discussed between the physician and the staff.

In these cases, the staff defined the situation as an ethical dilemma for both the patient and themselves, and in both cases they viewed the attending physician as uncaring and unethical. This perception continued because there was no input from the physician to indicate otherwise. The staff felt that they were put in the position of following orders or a request with which they disagreed and that, when they questioned the orders and the request, they were dissatisfied with the answer they received. The ethical problem with the patient remained, and they felt that the physician was not interested in the ethics of the case or in the staff's concerns.

In my role as consultant, it is important to know whether staff members feel that, as employees of the institution, their job security is threatened when they raise ethical issues and question the attending physician. If a staff member's job is at stake, how and where would she or he receive support if needed? When the case is complex, should I (1) contact the clinical ethics committee, (2) suggest that a staff member do this, or (3) urge the staff to reach some solution without involving the committee?

Although my position at this institution is an unsalaried clinical appointment, it is not clear to whom and in what way I am accountable while involved in these cases. An ethics consultation is an informal activity in that it does not activate any part of the bureaucracy. However, taking a case to the clinical ethics committee shifts the case into the formal structure of the institution. Therefore, the question of whether to keep the case on the unit or to contact the committee is a question of whether or not to bring a particular case into the formal structure of the institution.

In addition to discussing the ethics of a given case, it seems necessary to discuss potential strategies. In consulting with the 88 percent of caregivers who are not physicians but who have employee status in a complex, hierarchically ordered bureaucracy, it is unethical not to discuss strategies. But which strategies can and should be discussed and used by staff? Should the alternative of not following orders (or nonparticipation) be discussed and, if so, how will this influence the clinical world of patients and staff? The staff members have an obligation to the patients, but they need to know how they can best meet this obligation. At the same time, there is a duty to the physician to see that orders are carried out and that the patient receives the best care possible. What is the best care; by whose definition; and on the basis of what criteria? In each case in which I have been involved, this has been the underlying problem, coupled with the fact that the staff place the patient at the center of the ethical dilemma and define the physician as the major problem.

There are several other questions which an ethics consultant must raise. For example, to what extent should the ethics consultant adhere to ethical principles and theory in the questions I ask, and to what extent should these principles and theories be made explicit during a consultation? The consultation session with the staff, who are seldom entirely free from patient care duties, usually lasts up to an hour and a half. Since it is often a session in which people must come and go, it becomes quite complicated in terms of interaction and dynamics. It is less than an ideal time to try to teach ethical principles and theories to staff members.

SUMMARY

Ethical problems, issues, questions, and stances usually occur in a social context, and that context can have constraints that make raising questions and taking a stance a complex matter. The physician has a special legal and ethical relationship with the patient. The nurse has obligations to the patient, the institution, and the physician. The simple-minded answer to this situation is for nurses to act according to the American Nurses Association Code for Nurses. But life and ethical issues are sufficiently complicated that the code can only give the most general guidelines for action. An examination of these ethical problems with the 88 percent of nonphysician caregivers brings into sharp focus the fact that ethical dilemmas are not easily resolved and that there are numerous factors that must be considered in the reasoning process. Anyone acting as an ethics consultant with this group of institutional employees must not only have some basis in ethics and bioethics but also in the sociology of ethical decision making in these complex institutions.

Although in some instances nurses might not perceive ethical problems, there are also times when they deliberately choose not to see an ethical problem so that they will not have to confront it. This says much about the climate and morale of health care institutions.

REFERENCES

1. Prescott, Patricia R., and Brown, Sally A. "Physician-Nurse Relationship." *Annals of Internal Medicine* 103 (1985): 127–33.
2. Makadon, Harvey J., and Gibbons, M. Patricia. "Nurses and Physicians: Prospects for Collaboration." *Annals of Internal Medicine* 103 (1985): 134–36.
3. Gramelspacher, Gregory P.; Howell, Joel D.; and Young, Mark J. "Perceptions of Ethical Problems by Nurses and Doctors." *Archives of Internal Medicine* 146 (1986): 577–78.
4. Wagley, Philip F. "Doctor's Orders." *Archives of Internal Medicine* 140 (1980): 1553–54.

7

Hiring a Hospital Ethicist

James F. Drane

With increasing frequency, courts are holding hospitals responsible for ethical decisions made within their walls.[1,2] Some state
statutes and federal regulations also require assurance that ethical issues arising in hospital care are handled by staff members
in a sensitive and defensible way.[3-5] Accrediting agencies are
also looking closely at the way ethical decisions are made in
hospitals and at the policies that are in place to encourage
responsible decision-making procedures.[6] Both the federal government and professional associations have recommended hospital ethics committees to foster consultation and deliberation
when life-and-death decisions are made by surrogates or when
policies are implemented to address other sensitive issues such
as do-not-resuscitate orders.[7]

All of these developments mean that physicians and other
hospital staff members need training in ethics. Professional
groups have recognized this need and are now requiring ethics
and humanities courses as part of their training programs.[8]
Ethical questions are even appearing on certification examinations for certain specialties.[9] However, it will take some time
before these changes result in perceptible improvements in ethical decision-making procedures within specific institutions. In
the meantime, serious ethical dilemmas trouble practicing professionals in every hospital, and administrators may want to
take action to address them.

THE HOSPITAL ETHICIST

One solution for bridging the gap between current ethical needs of institutions and the availability of trained professionals to meet these needs is simply to hire a hospital ethicist. This additional staff member could be responsible for the ethics education of older staff members, provide ethics consultations, and serve on newly formed ethics committees. Such a person could be employed on either a full- or part-time basis.

There are many trained persons who are anxious to work in a clinical rather than an educational setting.[10] However, not all medical ethicists are suitable for hospital work. Hospital administrators would be well advised to look carefully at candidates before deciding to add an ethicist to the staff. The ethics education of doctors and nurses is a delicate and difficult task, and this challenge cannot be met by everyone who holds a Ph.D. degree. Some graduate-level education in philosophy and ethics involves high-flying metaphysical abstractions, and someone trained in such a way would be out of place in a hospital setting. Practicing doctors and nurses are used to continuing education requirements, but they insist that education be directly relevant to the many problems they face in patient care. It is not easy to organize classes and seminars around specific clinical issues, to find practical and understandable readings, and to maintain the interest of working people who have to squeeze ethics education into an already crowded schedule. Teaching doctors and nurses in a hospital setting is a bigger challenge than teaching the typical undergraduate on a university campus.

Aside from the added challenge of clinically based education, there are some extraordinary obstacles to be overcome by a staff ethicist. Many of the physicians with whom a hospital ethicist will work will think of medical ethics either as "fluff" or as a passing fad. They belong to the no-nonsense, tough-minded wing of the medical community and believe that problems in contemporary medicine can best be solved through continued scientific endeavor. The only acceptable ethical code for these doctors is the old ethic of professional competency:

The "good" doctor is one who knows what he is doing and works within the limits of his technical competency. According to these doctors, no "nonmedical expert" can improve the ethical atmosphere within a hospital, and they will be continually critical of a staff bioethicist.

Until recently, these tough-minded doctors constituted a majority. However, opinion has shifted in the past five years, and a new "tender-minded" approach has definitely gained ground. According to this "softer" model, the good doctor must be able to communicate with patients, be sensitive to patient values, encourage patient participation in treatment decisions, and generally be able to engage the whole person of the patient rather than just the patient's biological dimension. To comply with minimal legal requirements, a doctor must know how to obtain a valid informed consent and be able to communicate successfully with patients about treatment options.[11] Because more nonscientific skills are required to earn the designation "good" or "ethical" in this expanded sense, it seems logical to these "softer-minded" doctors to have an ethicist on the hospital staff who can help with the many ethical dimensions of modern clinical practice. Some, though not many, of the medical staff will welcome a clinical ethicist and be supportive to the point of joining study groups or leading small group discussions associated with clinical courses.

ETHICAL COMPETENCY AMONG PHYSICIANS

The expanded idea of the good doctor is endorsed by many medical leaders who have the power to reshape the educational process in medicine. They want doctors themselves to be capable of improved ethical decision making, and they encourage the addition of ethics training in medical school and residency programs.[12] The American Board of Internal Medicine, for example, requires that a physician show "integrity, respect, and compassion" before receiving board certification.[13] A list of new requirements was sent to the directors of 430 internal medicine residency programs, as well as to medical school deans and other physician-certifying boards. New physicians who fail to meet the more humanistic standards of professional behavior simply will not be licensed, and older doctors will not be recertified.

What type of behavior is considered essential to good practice, according to the new standards? The internal medicine board lists integrity and honesty in dealing with patients as one of its demands. This marks an interesting change, since previous ethical codes paid little or no attention to the value of truth or the virtue of honesty. Not telling the truth was so common among physicians in ancient Greece that even Plato thought that lying was acceptable for physicians.[14] It is hard to imagine that the standard medical ethics education will improve the character of physicians, but it could provide important information about just what should be disclosed to patients to ensure an informed consent and how to avoid the worst forms of patient abuse.

Aside from honesty, both ethics and the law now require the physician to respect patient choices and rights. Again, such respect has not been a prominent element in traditional medical codes.[15] In fact, for the "tough-minded" physician, the right to autonomy and patient participation in medical decision making is considered nothing but a nuisance created by lawyers meddling in medicine. They honor the informed consent requirement in only the most formalized way and, in substance, consider it impossible to achieve. But current American law, as well as professional ethical standards, have made old-style toughness both ethically wrong and legally dangerous. The doctor can and should make recommendations to the patient in an atmosphere of respect for patient preferences, which includes a careful disclosure of alternatives and options. Such an atmosphere can be created by better training in medical ethics, especially the ethical aspects of informed consent.

Finally, the good doctor, according to new standards of medical practice, must be able to show compassion and to recognize the special needs created by suffering and illness. Efficient manipulation of the tools of medicine is no longer enough. Because medical treatment involves human beings, humane responses are required of the treater. A comfort or compassion requirement is intended to eliminate abruptness, hostility, and generally insensitive communication. A physician can be trained to avoid uncompassionate behaviors and can learn to spend a few moments to touch the patient in a humane way. Characters will not be changed by having a clinical ethicist provide ethics courses for the staff, but a clinical ethics course could certainly include some concrete suggestions about how to approach patients concerning delicate issues, including what to say and how to communicate in a respectful way.

Leaders in the medical community are not alone in pushing for more attention to ethical and humanistic competencies among physicians. The U.S. government, and specifically the Department of Health and Human Services in the latest "Baby Doe" regulations, encourages attention to the ethical climate of health care institutions through the development of hospital committees, the first function of which is the ethics education of the staff.[16] Of course, physicians and nurses are important members of such committees, and their effective participation requires a new literacy in the discipline of ethics.

All of these changes make the addition of an ethicist to the hospital staff more plausible. The addition of one staff member can go a long way toward meeting new standards of practice and accomplishing important institutional goals. However, it would be a rare problem that could be solved simply by adding a new position. The right person must be found to fill the position, and the right kind of hospital ethicist is a person who is both well trained in ethics and familiar with the clinical setting. Most importantly, the right candidate is respectful of the experience of medical professionals and of the values of clinical medicine.[17]

RISKS OF EMPLOYING AN ETHICIST

Hiring an ethicist for hospital staff education, case consultation, and policy development carries some risks as well as possible benefits. A staff ethicist can do real mischief. Rather than helping to clarify issues, some ethicists may only add to the confusion. It may not be obvious, but there may be an informal system in place within the hospital for the resolution of ethical problems. Doctors may informally but consistently consult with one another and with nurses about situations that raise ethical questions. It may take more time than necessary, and it may not have the advantage of a formalized methodology, but patients and other professionals may consistently be consulted before arriving at ethically defensible decisions. "Muddling through" does not always produce bad decisions.

An ethicist, who is trained in a tradition other than medicine and who may be suspicious of a physician's power, may actually promote antimedical values under the banner of ethics. Ethics may provide a platform for negative criticism of medical research and practice. If, for example, the ethicist focuses exclusively on the patient advocacy aspects of his or her role, or is committed to the primacy of patient autonomy over patient welfare, then medical ethics is likely to become a source of disruption and conflict. Patient advocacy has a legitimate place in the hospital, and autonomy is certainly a key value, but the ethicist must be more than the official watchdog for patient rights.

Another risk is authoritarianism. Dictatorial and self-righteous behavior is inappropriate in any profession. No one profession has a corner on eternal ethical truths. If the physician is the professional who is primarily responsible for the patient, a medical ethicist with insight provided by the literary disciplines can offer help but cannot take over decision making or presume to tell the physician what to do. Medical discretion is rooted in medical experience, and both must be respected by anyone working in a clinical setting. What then is appropriate? In most cases, a hospital ethicist can provide a valuable service by clarifying the ethical issues generated by a particular case. In addition, there will certainly be situations in which the ethicist advocates one opinion over another, but he or she should only perform this service when asked and should do so without appearing to take charge of decision making or assuming an air of infallibility.

The issue of misplaced authority can take many different

forms. Some bioethicists delight in calling attention to the poverty of ethics education in medical schools. They draw the conclusion that physicians do not recognize value choices; that is, that doctors convert ethical issues into technical medical matters and act as though their decisions were strictly matters of medical expertise. There is a certain truth to this accusation. Many doctors do feel uncomfortable with the unwieldy bioethics literature and try to defend themselves against charges of ignorance by denying the applicability and relevance of ethical categories to medicine. In so doing, they reduce medical acts to purely technical maneuvers and convert medicine into a seemingly value-free activity.

But ethical reasoning is very much a part of medicine. Both doctors and patients constantly choose among options, and the choices are often based on personal interests, needs, and preferences rather than on objective scientific considerations. Those who distort medicine into a value-neutral, technical exercise turn all the many ethical elements within medicine into something different. By so doing, they make medical practice vulnerable to the harshest critics of medicine.

At the opposite extreme, some academically oriented ethicists hold a distorted conception of medicine because they see ethics as an immense nonmedical value territory within medical practice, and they look upon themselves as the experts in this territory. Paradoxically, this view turns ethics into just as narrow and distorted a field as that of purely technical medicine. Ethicists become narrow technical experts. A distorted concept of value-free medicine generates an equally distorted concept of ethics. Both medicine and ethics thereby become a matter for technicians, and both disciplines are depersonalized. Doctors who see medicine as a technical, value-free practice overlook the important ethical elements in their practice, and ethicists who see values in medicine as separate from the experience of doctors overlook the same ethical elements in clinical practice. The ethically insensitive physician is a dangerous member of a hospital staff, and the clinically insensitive ethicist is simply no help to a hospital.

One way to avoid the above-mentioned risks is to look for

a person who recognizes the ethical content in ordinary medical practice. He or she should have a deep respect for the essentially ethical structure of the doctor-patient relationship and for the traditional ethics of medicine. Even though they may have little formal ethical training, most doctors are thoroughly immersed in ethics. The committed physician is dedicated to caring for persons in need, and in all but the most routine cases physicians use ethical discretion. This means that they make choices based on what they believe is best for the patient; that is, ethics. Ethics does not arrive at the hospital when a bioethics expert is hired. Hospital ethicists who recognize the inherent ethics of ordinary medical practice and who respect this reality can contribute to the ethical atmosphere of the hospital, but someone whose only understanding of medical ethics is based on technical philosophy is a risk.

Administrators might be well advised to determine whether candidates for a hospital ethics position have clinical experience or at least some identification with medicine as a profession. Affirmative answers to both questions would not necessarily preclude a mistake but would create a favorable presumption. In addition, some direct questions about how candidates view their own field may be helpful. Is medical ethics primarily a body of technical information concerning rules and laws? Does the candidate see an inevitable struggle for authority in the hospital? How does the candidate view the ethical development of physicians? Is the lack of ethical development among physicians strictly a matter of the absence of formal ethics training? Is the ethicist the sole authority when it comes to the value areas of medicine? The answers to these questions will give the administrator a sense of what sort of ethicist is applying for work. It is difficult enough to manage a hospital full of medical authorities without introducing an opposing authority who has little respect for what doctors do.

CARRYING OUT THE HOSPITAL ETHICIST'S WORK

What kind of strategy would be most appropriate to the work of a hospital ethicist? Surely it is not abstract philosophizing or trying to clarify issues at their most abstract levels. Issues such as the nature of human freedom are important, and they certainly provide a good topic for a graduate seminar, but the exploration of broad, abstract issues is not ordinarily of much help to working members of the medical staff. This type of intellectual work is better done in more traditional university settings. The same is true of questions such as the nature of rights, the foundations of human responsibilities, and the intersection of science and technology with the humanities.

The staff ethicist ordinarily has to stay closer to concrete cases and to the goal of developing defensible decision-making strategies for particular cases. The practice of hospital medical ethics starts with and remains focused upon concrete life situations. What is the right thing to do for *this* comatose patient? Should the defective neonate born to the young unmarried mother be treated? What should be done with the seriously ill patient who is refusing treatment? Should treatment be forced in this case? How much should we tell the patient in Room 202 who is terrified of having cancer? How do we know whether the newly arrived patient is competent to refuse treatment?

To be useful in a hospital setting, an ethicist must first have a feel for the concrete clinical situation. He or she can help hospital staff members to develop the conceptual tools to think through cases and arrive at defensible ethical decisions. Concepts must be clarified, alternatives must be outlined, elements of a case structure must be considered, and the sensitive physician's inclinations must be taken into account. The ethicist who can do all of this unobtrusively represents the best risk/benefit ratio for a hospital staff position. Medical ethics so conceived and practiced stands the best chance of making a contribution to a health care institution struggling to provide better staff education in medical ethics and to improve the climate for sound ethical decision making within the institution.

Put more specifically, a good hospital ethicist should be able to help physicians recognize the ubiquitous moral dimensions of even ordinary medical practice. Sensational cases may be interesting, but to focus exclusively on these suggests that ethics is a rare rather than an omnipresent aspect of practice. As a matter of fact, every patient encounter and every medical act has its ethical dimensions. For example, the communication between doctor and patient has everything to do with whether the patient gets adequate information, understands his or her options, and finally gives an ethically valid consent. Good hospital ethicists should be able to help the hospital staff to provide all that is required for a truly informed consent.

As a member of a health care team, the ethicist should understand and be able to explain: the meaning of terms such as "patient competence"; when refusal of treatment ordinarily occurs; what options the clinician has in the face of such refusals; ways of avoiding litigation by negotiating consent with the patient, the family, and the physician; different concepts of death and how brain death differs from persistent vegetative state; how suicide is distinguished from refusal of risky treatment; the difference between direct and indirect killing; the interpretations of "slippery slope"; surrogate decision making; the dying process; the physician's privilege to withhold information in certain cases; the limits of confidentiality; and equitable distribution of health care.

Not unlike the good teacher, a hospital ethicist's command of the conceptual issue must be complemented by good interactional skills. In addition to being able to teach certain skills, hospital ethicists will frequently be asked to use them themselves. Some hospital cases will require mediation by a nonmedical person, and the ethicist may be the indicated mediator. Families may need assurance that the doctors are doing all they can or that the family decision about withholding treatment is an altogether appropriate one. Parents may need help in coming to a decision about a defective infant. The hospital ethicist might help in all of these areas. The hospital ethicist may also have to run some small group seminars as part of an interdisciplinary committee and may have to chair a committee or two.

Since the hospital ethicist will often be consulted about sensitive issues by doctors with highly developed egos, he or she will have to provide help without appearing to dictate solutions. The ability to do this is no small personal skill. The hospital is no place for a power-hungry ethicist or one who is socially withdrawn.

INTERVIEWING THE APPLICANT

A well-structured interview can provide quite a bit of insight into the personality of a job applicant. The hospital administrator ought to be able to identify socially introverted personalities, as well as those who are outgoing but essentially narcissistic. In addition to these obvious personal traits, there are other attitudes, leanings, and dispositions that ought to be assessed. Administrators should avoid applicants who are:

1. *Too theoretical.* Hospital administrators should ensure that the candidate for hospital ethicist is not too strongly wedded to metaethical theory. Theory is important, indeed embedded in every form of praxis, but in the hospital setting, negotiating the settlement of a conflict may be more important than theoretical purity. The best course of action in a particular clinical setting may be more accurately dictated by an experienced doctor's discretion than by a deontological or utilitarian theory of right and wrong.

2. *Dogmatic.* A clinical setting is a place of compromise and no place for a person who suffers from moral inflexibility.

3. *Obsessive/compulsive.* The perfectly right thing can seldom be done in the hospital, and it cannot be done immediately. Decisions about difficult cases are often made by "muddling along" until an ethically defensible solution emerges.

4. *Too directive.* More than one set of interests often intersect in the clinical setting; the ethicist must take into account the interests of the doctors, the nurses, the patients, and the hospital administration. He or she cannot dictate the right course of action. Mediation is often more important than direction.

5. *Too aggressive*. No hospital needs a "wimp" for an ethicist, but a strong ethicist must have good mediation skills. It is not a sign of weakness for the ethicist to avoid striking back in the face of hostility.

6. *Too paternalistic*. Good clinical ethicists do not insist on what they think is best for others, but they should be sympathetic to the paternalism that is part of good care in many institutional settings. Doctors and nurses in acute care settings, especially those in long-term care facilities, must help people decide what is best for them, a soft form of paternalism.

7. *Too literalistic*. The good clinical ethicist must have some psychiatric sophistication, showing sensitivity to the deeper dimensions of what people say rather than dealing with only the most literal meaning of discourse.

Aside from having the right personality characteristics, the applicant must know something about bioethics. The hospital administrator who is not conversant with the field should look for familiarity with certain concepts and content.

Professional persons give some indication of their qualifications by familiarity with the literature of the field. Modern medical ethics is not an old field, but already the literature has expanded beyond the capacities of even the most efficient and avid reader. The competent clinical ethicist should be familiar with certain basic resources. The standard journals include the *Hastings Center Report*, the *Journal of Bioethics*, the *Journal of Medicine and Philosophy*, the *Journal of the American Medical Association*, and the *New England Journal of Medicine*. The Kennedy Institute at Georgetown University and the Hastings Center at Briarcliff, New York are the two major research facilities in the field. A candidate should certainly know about both of these centers and be familiar with the work of these ethicists, who have authored a great deal of the current literature: Robert M. Veatch, H. Tristram Engelhardt, Jr., Tom L. Beauchamp, Richard A. McCormick, Daniel Callahan, Paul Ramsey, James Rachels, George Annas, William May, Edmund Pellegrino, and James Childress. This list obviously is not presumed to be exhaustive.

Because certain themes persist in the literature, it may be helpful to ask an applicant about them; for example, about the difference between procedural and normative issues or between who should decide (procedural) and the right or wrong thing to do (normative). Likewise, moral principles, such as autonomy and beneficence, should be familiar, and any applicant should be able to provide examples of how these principles operate in clinical situations. Certain legal cases have had a major impact on the field of bioethics; all applicants should be familiar with the Quinlan, Saikewicz, Dinnerstein, Baby Doe, Baby Jane Doe, Conroy, and Brophy cases. Applicants should be questioned about the above-mentioned distinctions and principles in the context of the major legal cases. In the Quinlan case, for example, there was a question about whether the physicians or the family should make decisions about withdrawing treatment (the procedural question). The ethicist should be able to distinguish between who had the right to decide (the procedural issue) and what was the right thing to do for Karen Ann (the normative question). The same questions arose in the case of Baby Jane Doe, the New York baby with severe birth defects.

SPECIAL INSTITUTIONAL NEEDS

Because hospitals are not all the same, not every administrator will want the same competencies in a staff ethicist. A sophisticated university-based facility or large teaching hospital may want an ethicist who is able to swim in deeper intellectual waters. Because bioethics does not exist as a totally separate discipline, but has developed out of the larger moral context called the "culture of medicine," historical changes in medicine have changed the moral context in which medicine is practiced, thereby changing the nature of the ethics of medicine. This subtle interaction between medical ethics and the practice of medicine is a higher-level epistemological issue, and not every administrator will be interested in having an ethicist who has a grasp of issues at this level. In an academic hospital, however, such an interest and competency may be an important qualification.

If the administrator is responsible for an institution that is known for its teaching and houses a whole range of residency programs, he or she may be interested in how much experience an applicant has had with nontraditional teaching and learning. An ethicist who has successfully developed creative ways of teaching may be more attractive than one who has a grasp of the history of medicine or the subtle interplay between ethics and forms of medical practice. Asking for suggestions about nontraditional approaches to ethics education for clinical professionals would provide some important information about the applicant.

Another institution may be facing very difficult economic and social issues. A very specialized type of medical ethicist would be required if, for example, a Catholic hospital system with a long history of effective management of clinical ethical issues were suddenly faced with a host of questions about equity, justice, and economic security. Such a hospital system, and the religious order that runs it, may historically have been committed to caring for the poor and may now see itself competing for the health care dollar with aggressive for-profit hospital chains. There are experts in the social and economic aspects of medical ethics and specialists in the many new forms of health care delivery. Most likely, however, the ordinary applicant for a staff ethicist position would not be very helpful with such questions, although they arise in many institutions today and certainly qualify as a dimension of contemporary medical ethics.

There are highly specialized institutions, too, that need a highly specialized ethicist. Genetic experimentation and its application to human reproduction are both shot through with difficult ethical problems. Advances in genetic medicine have given us new visions of human possibility, and choosing from among these visions is certainly an ethical enterprise. Some medical ethicists specialize in genetic issues, and they could be of great help to an institution where important genetic research and treatment is taking place. Throughout most of history, medicine could do little about infertility and inherited disease. During that same time, medicine did not have much of an impact on human society, certainly not on the very image of humanness in society. But now medicine has the potential to change everything, and the medical ethics of the future are different from the discipline that we have been discussing. It is much more involved with social goods and philosophical visions. An institution that is pioneering this future reality will need a highly specialized ethicist.

The substantive reality of genetic research and the future roles of medicine in society are issues that are very far removed from the mass media's superficial fascination with medical ethics. If a hospital hires an ethicist, that person may be expected to have contact with the media about certain cases. Given such a possibility, the administrator may want to set down some guidelines for interaction with the media and to examine the applicant's ability to represent the hospital in a judicious way. If the administrator intends for the hospital ethicist to make himself or herself available to the media (to reassure an even more cynical public about the hospital's commitment to human values), then certain obvious talents and experience will be required.

CONCLUSION

If there is one central point in this chapter, it is that the hospital ethicist must be sensitive to the peculiarities of a clinical setting and respectful of persons with extensive clinical experience. A few examples will support this point.

Certain problems are associated with members of the clergy who minister to people, and there are problems within the institutions that train the clergy. The minister, priest, or rabbi, like the doctor, is a professional who exercises power. As in medicine, there is an ever-present possibility of doing good or harm through the use of that power. The doctor is not the only one who can do either great good or great harm, and medicine is not the only profession whose members face ethical dilemmas.

But suppose someone suggested that an outside expert be brought in to instruct both the faculty and the seminary students about ethics. How do you think that suggestion would be met? Probably not very well. Once the shock of disbelief was overcome, the arguments against any such idea are easy to imagine. "Only those who have experience in the ministry, who face the problems, who exercise the power, and who have suffered remorse from mistakes, can presume to talk with authority about ethics in ministry." "Only those on the inside can be the primary ethicists of ministry." An outside expert who knows how professions tend to form a person's view of reality, as well as how they form members for the task at hand, could admittedly be helpful — but not with the concrete practical dilemmas facing the clergy. The primary ethicists for ministry, the faculty and students would argue, would have to be clerics, persons with clerical experience who actually exercise clerical power.

Take academic life as another example. There are numerous ethical problems within the university, many of which are rooted in the exercise of power. The case of a young psychologist at the University of California who had sexual relations with many of his students provided a good example of ethical abuse stemming from misuse of the real power of a teacher over students. He was using that power for his own benefit and passing off his private indulgence as some sort of educational experience. What he did was unethical, and there are all sorts of other examples one could cite of structural and individual immorality within the university. But suppose it was suggested that outside experts be brought in to teach ethics to teachers. Do you think anyone would attend the lectures? And how would an academic staff ethicist be treated by professional colleagues? Great benefit could be derived from attention to ethical issues in the context of teaching, but those with the experience must be the first ones to recognize the issues and to take the first steps toward change.

There is little doubt that a medical ethicist could be a helpful addition to a hospital staff. Because physicians today must take many more variables into account to make ethically sound and legally defensible decisions, some continuing training in ethics should be made available in hospitals. Ethics grand rounds would be a helpful part of the hospital's continuing education program. Residency training programs and nursing programs within the hospital must also include formal medical ethics training. An on-staff ethicist could provide these services in addition to serving on ethics committees. Many groups within the hospital need professional input from a trained ethicist to carry out their clinical functions.

The need for a medical ethicist in the modern hospital, especially a teaching hospital or medical center, is real and obvious. The right kind of medical ethicist for a particular institution is not so obvious. There is good reason to be careful in making the selection.

NOTES

1. Edward E. Hollowell, "Does Hospital Corporate Liability Extend to Medical Staff Supervision?" *Medical and Health Care* 101 (1982): 225.
2. The *Quinlan* decision provided strong support for the ethics committee requirements. *In re Quinlan*, 70 N.F. 10, 335 A.2d 647 (1976).
3. Pennsylvania Department of Health, General and Special Hospitals, "Patient's Bill of Rights," *Pennsylvania Bulletin* 10 (September 20, 1980): 3761, 3676 S 103.22 (8) (9).
4. President's Commission for the Study of Ethical Problems in Medicine and Biomedical and Behavioral Research, *Deciding to Forego Life-Sustaining Treatment* (Washington, DC: U.S. Government Printing Office, 1982).
5. Baby Doe Regulations, 45 Code of Federal Regulations 1340, *Federal Register* (1985): 14878–901.
6. Joint Commission on Accreditation of Hospitals. *Accreditation Manual for Hospitals* (Chicago: Joint Commission on Accreditation of Hospitals, 1981).
7. President's Commission, *Deciding to Forego Life-Sustaining Treatment*.
8. Thomas K. McElhinney, *Human Values Teaching Programs for Health Professionals* (Ardmore, PA: Whitmore Publishing Co., 1981).
9. American Board of Internal Medicine. *A Guide to Awareness and Eval-*

uation of Humanistic Qualities in the Internists (Philadelphia, PA: American Board of Internal Medicine, 1985).

10. For a list of programs that train medical ethicists, see Doris Mueller Goldstein, *Bioethics: A Guide to Information Sources* (Detroit: Gale Research Co., 1982).

11. President's Commission for the Study of Ethical Problems in Medicine and Biomedical and Behavioral Research, "The Law of Informed Consent," in *Making Health Care Decisions* (Washington, DC: U.S. Government Printing Office, 1982), 193–246.

12. Jo Boufford, "The Teaching of Humanities and Health Values in Primary Care Residency Training: An Effort Begins," *Family Medicine* 14 (1982).

13. American Board of Internal Medicine, *A Guide to Awareness and Evaluation of Humanistic Qualities in the Internists*.

14. Bok, Sissela. "Truth Telling: Ethical Aspects," in *Encyclopedia of Bioethics*, ed. Warren T. Reich (New York: Free Press, 1978), 1677–88.

15. For a list of codes and statements related to medical ethics, see *Encyclopedia of Bioethics*, ed. Warren T. Reich (New York: Free Press, 1978). A new AMA code was approved in 1980.

16. Baby Doe Regulations, 45 Code of Federal Regulations 1340.

17. James F. Drane, *Becoming a Good Doctor: The Place of Virtue and Character in Medical Ethics* (Kansas City, Sheed & Ward, 1988). This book, written for physicians, discusses the character traits mentioned by the American Board of Internal Medicine.

Part III

Values

INTRODUCTION

Ethical problems are inherently controversial and involve conflicting values or principles. Ethics consultants have ethical biases that move them to favor certain types of resolutions to conflict. Can consultants monitor their own biases? What kinds of help can institutions offer to "watch the ethicists" for favoritism or bias?

Part III has two chapters that are responsive to these questions. Edmund G. Howe, whose work combines psychiatry, ethics, and law, examines five types of cases in which physicians tend to impose their biases on patients. These are (1) cases in which patients have poor prognoses but desire full treatment, (2) cases which involve a determination of competency, (3) cases which involve protection from legal liability, (4) cases which require protection of third parties from patients with AIDS, and (5) cases which require a consideration of benefit to patients' families.

Albert R. Jonsen recalls a case in which an elderly woman refused a life-sustaining surgical procedure. Drawing on this case, he raises questions about the source of authority for ethics consultation, the legal status of his advice, the place of ethics consultation in the quality of care provided in hospitals, and whether he should have intervened at all in the situation.

8

When Physicians Impose Values on Patients: An Ethics Consultant's Responsibilities

Edmund G. Howe

New medical technology has made it possible to prolong some patients' lives indefinitely. In cases where this treatment is futile and does not benefit the patient, it is often viewed as prolonging death rather than life and, accordingly, courts have made it easier for patients to have treatment withheld or withdrawn. Greater scarcity of resources and the emergence of acquired immune deficiency syndrome (AIDS) have also presented new situations in which physicians may, wittingly or unwittingly, impose personal values on patients.

The ethics consultant has several options when confronting these situations. This chapter focuses on one particularly critical option, whether the ethics consultant should assert a definitive position and insist that others adopt his position or remain more neutral, primarily clarifying alternatives. The former approach is more likely to protect an individual patient's immediate interests in the short run, but it may alienate the physician and deprive the ethics consultant of opportunities to help a greater number of patients in the long run.

Five types of situations in which physicians might impose biases will be considered: when treating patients who have

This paper represents the view of the author only and in no way reflects the views of the Uniformed Services University of the Health Sciences or the Department of Defense.

poor prognoses but desire full treatment; when determining patients' competency and "subjective" interests; when protecting themselves or their institution from legal liability; when protecting third parties from patients with AIDS; and when attempting to benefit patients' families.

It is argued that physicians have a strong obligation to further patient interests in the first three situations, but that it does not necessarily follow that the ethics consultant should become the patient's advocate. Instead, the marked moral superiority of one approach and general consensus that this superiority exists are minimal (if insufficient) criteria for an ethics consultant to assert a patient's interests even over and against the interests of the referring physician. Finally, when an ethical consensus exists, the ethics consultant may accomplish more, at least initially, by sharing this consensus and its basis than by presenting his or her own views. The existence of consensus itself implies that its reasons are compelling, whereas the ethics consultant's views may be perceived as idiosyncratic beliefs.

PATIENTS WITH POOR PROGNOSES

Traditional medical ethics holds that the physician's first obligation is to the patient. Exceptions to this principle involve such cases as gunshot wounds, sexually transmitted diseases, and child abuse, but spiralling medical costs and limited resources have recently challenged this priority. When the government cannot make dialysis available to patients in Britain, for example, physicians may not inform these patients that dialysis could be immensely beneficial.[1] These physicians may be seen as serving the interests of the government, not their patients.

Physicians in the United States often give priority to one patient (or to society's interests) over another patient.[2] When, for example, two patients ideally should be admitted to an intensive care unit (ICU), but only one bed is available, physicians have reported that, if one patient is considerably older than the other, they inform the older patient that while he or she may choose to enter the ICU, it will be in the place of a younger patient who stands to benefit by living more years. These physicians justify this practice on the principle of truth-telling, but acknowledge that they are also furthering their bias in favor of the younger patient's interests.

This approach elicits older patients' guilt and, even if they choose to be admitted to the ICU, it directly harms them. The physician is balancing the older patients' interests against those of younger patients and is, therefore, violating the trust upon which the doctor-patient relationship is founded.

Doctors in some hospitals decide which of two patients to transfer to an ICU on an almost daily basis.[3] If they fail to inform patients when they make decisions on this basis, they implicitly deceive them, because the patient believes the physician is acting in his or her interest. If transfer to another hospital cannot be accomplished, a physician could defer these decisions to a "neutral" decision maker or withdraw from cases in which patients' interests conflict. If a decision must be made, unless the doctor favors a paternalistic approach to this situation, the patients should know the basis of these decisions.

Some physicians go further to preserve staff resources or save society money by actively discouraging terminally ill patients from choosing treatments which would prolong their lives. The physicians describe to patients in disturbing detail, for example, the worst circumstances which could result after they are resuscitated (such as becoming dependent upon a respirator and beset by pain which cannot be controlled by drugs) to "convince" these patients to request do-not-resuscitate orders. This behavior is deceitful because it selects one possible outcome and implies that this is the only or most probable outcome. Legally, frightening patients so that they refuse beneficial treatments may represent negligent overdisclosure of information.

DETERMINING PATIENT COMPETENCY

Theoretically, incompetency is a legal determination which must always be decided by a court. In practice, however, judicial declarations are not always sought. Some physicians assert that if declarations of incompetency were sought for all patients whose competence was questionable, doctors who work with such patients would spend all their time in court.

Patients who accept treatment which is beneficial are often treated in spite of questionable competency, especially if family members agree with the treatment being given. Generally, when a patient who may be incompetent refuses treatment, physicians are advised to consult a psychiatrist.

Like the physician, however, the psychiatrist may unwittingly impose his or her own value biases when determining competency. In many jurisdictions, psychiatrists can choose the standard for competency they wish to apply.[4] They may only require that a patient literally understand his or her alternatives; or they may require that the patient understand the alternatives well enough to manipulate this information. If the psychiatrist chooses the former standard, it is more likely that the patient will be judged competent than if he uses the latter, stricter standard.

The psychiatrist or physician may unwittingly impose a bias by placing inordinate significance on those clinical findings which support his or her value preference, especially when the stricter standard is used. A physician supported his bias in this manner, for example, when a patient who was dying of cancer expressed his wish to marry his fiancée before his death. This patient's cancer had metastasized to his brain so that his mental status fluctuated between periods of lucidity and confusion. His physician deemed him incompetent to make this decision on the basis of these fluctuations, and obstructed the patient's taking measures to fulfill his desire. During a lucid period the patient affirmed that he knew he would probably die in the very near future, but he still wanted to get married. When asked why he wished to get married under these circumstances, his face expressed incredulity. "Because I love her," he simply responded.

The physician later acknowledged that, in fact, he had judged this patient incompetent because he wished to prevent the patient's fiancée from receiving monetary compensation from the patient's employer after the patient died. Whether or not the physician was right in deeming the patient incompetent is open to question. This patient was wholly dependent on the environment supporting him and his capacity to make a truly autonomous choice may have been substantially impaired. Nonetheless, this example illustrates how, when determining a patient's competency, a physician or psychiatrist can select data to support his or her own values.

Similarly, physicians can impose their own bias when they serve on ethics committees and are asked to determine an incompetent patient's "subjective preference." This standard is intended to respect such patients' dignity by enabling surrogate decision makers to identify their individual needs and preferences as accurately as possible. These goals were exemplified in the case of Joseph Saikewicz, who was 67 years old, had an IQ of ten, and had been institutionalized for his entire life. After this patient developed acute myeloblastic monocytic leukemia, caregivers feared that, if given chemotherapy, he would misinterpret their actions and believe they were mistreating him. Though the average person would have wanted chemotherapy, the chemotherapy was withheld.[5]

Yet, when Mary Hier, a 92-year-old woman, stopped taking thorazine and ripped out her gastrostomy tube, caregivers questioned whether the tube should be surgically reinserted. One surgeon stated that he believed this patient's subjective preference was that she wanted to die. Subsequently he, like the physician who deemed his patient incompetent to get married, acknowledged that he had expressed this opinion primarily because he believed that providing further treatment to this patient would waste society's money.[6]

PHYSICIANS' LEGAL INTERESTS VERSUS PATIENTS' MEDICAL INTERESTS

Instances in which physicians have placed their own legal interests above those of patients are notorious. Until a new army regulation was adopted,[7] for example, it was the policy of one military hospital to have physicians writing do-not-resuscitate (DNR) orders to note in the chart that the nurse should contact the physician on call in the event of cardiopulmonary arrest. A civilian hospital placed decals on the charts of patients who had DNR orders and removed them after these patients died.[8] The use of these euphemisms, however, is not what has harmed patients. The source of harm is physicians' beliefs that patients or their surrogate decision makers should not, under any circumstances, be given DNR orders.

Some doctors have attempted to protect themselves legally by ordering verbal "slow" codes (an agreement to be slow about calling a code in the event of cardiac or respiratory arrest) when they believed that patients would be better off dying, or that their dying would save staff or society's resources. Despite the American Heart Association's and the ethical and legal communities' clear opposition to slow codes,[9] this practice persists in some institutions. Even in places where it has been abandoned, equivalent measures (such as an abbreviated code or the "chemical" code in which usual drugs are not given) have taken its place.

Some physicians defend these practices, claiming that stopping a code is a judgment call anyway and that these practices represent no deviation from customary practice. It could be argued that physicians must exercise discretion on an ad hoc basis if patients' and their families' individual needs are to be met. Yet serious harm can result from physicians exercising such discretion. Doctors' views also vary widely concerning which additional interventions should be withheld when a do-not-resuscitate order has been written.[10] Because a DNR order had been written, a physician ordered a nurse to stop suctioning a patient who was choking from secretions; yet suffocation is an agonizing way to die.

In most of the situations just described, the exploitation of or harm to the patient is clear, and there is general ethical consensus that the physicians' behaviors are not justified. Under these two conditions, the ethics consultant has a strong prima facie obligation to advocate the patients' interests. Nonetheless, this obligation may be overridden. Whether or not the ethics consultant insists that the physician follow this position may depend on many additional factors, such as the likelihood that this would preclude the opportunity to help other patients in the future, the institutional support the ethics consultant is likely to receive, and the expectations and flexibility of the physician who requested the consultation.

As a practical matter, the ethics consultant may lose credibility if he or she does not assert a strong position when these two conditions are present. On the other hand, an effective ethics consultant should stress the existence and rationale of the ethical consensus rather than his or her personal view, though both are in agreement. Physicians will be less likely to perceive the consultant as attempting to impose his or her idiosyncratic bias and more likely to focus on the reasoning behind that position.

If, on the other hand, only one or neither of the above criteria is present, as illustrated by the situations which follow, the superiority of the ethics consultant's moral preferences is considerably more suspect. The ethics consultant's approach might well differ accordingly.

PROTECTING THIRD PARTIES FROM PATIENTS WHO HAVE AIDS OR HIV-RELATED ILLNESS

Physicians treating patients with AIDS and other HIV-related diseases sometimes must decide whether or not to place third parties' interests ahead of those of their patients. If, for example, such patients are unwilling to tell their spouses or intimate friends about their disease, physicians may consider violating their patients' confidentiality to inform these third parties. Some physicians have also considered trying to commit patients with HIV when they believe these patients will continue to be promiscuous.

The physician may have an obligation to warn a specific party in danger, particularly if there is a high probability of harm. On the other hand, committing a patient under these circumstances may represent preventative detention, which is unconstitutional in the United States.

Notwithstanding the absence of direct legal precedents,

one caregiver informed a patient with HIV that unless the patient informed his partner about his illness, he would violate this patient's confidentiality, because he would prefer being sued for breaking his patient's confidentiality than by the patient's partner after she acquired HIV. Since physicians are not required to report positive tests for HIV in many states, it would appear that there is no ethical consensus on how physicians should approach these situations. The ethics consultant's own preference may reflect his or her personal bias. It might be best to present the options and, when stating his or her opinion, suggest the possibility that it may represent inadvertent bias. Otherwise, the consultant may risk losing credibility with the referring physician.

Still, in some situations, an AIDS patient's interests may override the third party's interests. A question which arose for military physicians, for example, was whether or not they should warn active duty patients prior to taking a sexual history that they would report admissions of homosexuality to the officials. A regulation subsequently adopted protects soldiers in this situation.[11] Prior to this regulation, a soldier with HIV who reported previous homosexual activity could be discharged administratively and lose medical benefits. Three navy patients with HIV were administratively discharged after divulging homosexuality to navy physicians who reported them.[12]

Without giving any warning, these physicians used their medical role to induce these patients to incriminate themselves, and violated their implicit promise to put these patients' interests first. There is general ethical consensus that patients' vulnerability should not be exploited in this manner, unless the consequences of not doing so are extraordinary. Conceivably, the latter criterion is met in this circumstance. If not, the argument for the ethics consultant's advocating on these patients' behalf is much stronger.

PROTECTING PATIENTS' FAMILIES

When a patient with a terminal illness asks his physician not to inform his family, a physician who agrees to this request also implicitly agrees to deceive the patient's family. Two army regulations require that army physicians respect patients' confidentiality when patients request that a do-not-resuscitate order be written[13] or that treatment be withheld or withdrawn without their family being informed.[14]

To consider the potential harmful consequences of the first request only, if the family were visiting when the patient arrested and had not been informed that the patient had a DNR order, they would cry out for help and only then be told of the patient's request. This scene actually occurred when Rose Dreyer, an 87-year-old woman, had a cardiac arrest after having been given a DNR order without her relatives being informed. The grandson, a physician, was visiting at the time, and the hospital is now being sued for $20 million.[15]

Physicians have other options when confronting either situation. Physicians could, for instance, establish a ward policy to inform relatives of patients whose medical condition might warrant these requests that, in the event that patients make these requests and wish to keep them confidential, the patients' wishes would be respected. If such a ward policy could not be implemented, the physician could tell a patient that he or she cannot provide treatment under these circumstances or that this request could only be honored if the physician can also tell the family that the confidentiality of any patient making this request would be respected. This latter approach would alert the family to this possibility. These approaches are untraditional and coercive, but they maximize the likelihood that the patient and family will discuss the patient's decision meaningfully. They also free the physician from having to deceive the family.

Physicians encountering these situations may feel ambivalent about having to deceive these families by respecting these patients' requests. The ethics consultant might therefore inquire what weight physicians believe they can give their moral values under these and other circumstances. Physicians may not consider this possibility because they place such priority on meeting patients' needs. One cardiac surgeon, for example, was asked by a Jehovah's Witness patient to perform cardiac surgery without using blood and without informing his family. The physician was willing to perform the operation but had moral qualms about not telling the family. He had never considered offering to perform the operation on the condition that the patient tell his family.

The ethics consultant might remind physicians that the law permits them to refuse to perform acts they consider immoral, such as abortion. The ethics consultant should also point out, however, that while the physician may use his or her own moral values as a shield, they can also be used as a sword to pressure patients into complying with the physician's beliefs. If the physician is coercive, the reasons should be explained to the patient. Only then can the physician respect both the patient and his or her own values.

When, as in the latter two situations, the relative merits of options are less certain and ethical consensus is more problematic, the ethics consultant should indicate that his or her personal preference may reflect a bias. This gesture will demonstrate for physicians that they too should consider their preferences suspect when the logic of their position is not self-evident or compelling and when ethical consensus or other authority is absent. By qualifying the validity of this ethical opinion, the ethics consultant also stays within his or her expertise and is likely to further the credibility of the consultant role.

CONCLUSION

The five situations presented in this chapter represent a spectrum in which patients' interests are more clearly violated on one hand and third parties' interests are violated on the other. In cases in which patients are more severely harmed, such as when they are deprived of life-sustaining means or when they are kept alive against their will, the ethics consultant will probably be compelled to be an advocate for the patients' interests. In other cases, in which the ethically preferable option is more equivocal, the ethics consultant may choose primarily to elucidate alternatives.

Some physicians, such as those who feel justified in pressuring patients to make choices to benefit other patients, may be totally unwilling to consider other points of view. The ethics consultant may take an adversarial position against such physicians or, if harm to the patient is minimal, may choose not to take a stand. If the ethics consultant acknowledges the particular merits of the physician's opposing view while clearly disagreeing with it, the physician may come around to the consultant's view.

Other physicians will be more open to options they had not previously considered, particularly if the options further values that are consistent with their previous value priorities. Physicians may, for example, want to protect third parties from patients with HIV and to protect patients' families from patients requesting confidentiality, because in both instances these physicians would be protecting potential victims from harm, a major tenet of the Hippocratic oath. The role of the ethics consultant in facilitating this decision would be to illuminate values that the physician had not seen in these cases.

Some believe that that is all an ethics consultant can do in any case. Regardless, the most effective ethics consultant will be the one who provides illumination rather than persuasion.

References

1. Schwartz, Robert, and Grubb, Andrew. "Why Britain Can't Afford Informed Consent." *Hastings Center Report* 15 (1985): 19–25.
2. Zawacki, Bruce E. "ICU Physician's Ethical Role in Distributing Scarce Resources." *Critical Care Medicine* 13 (1985): 57–60.
3. Zawacki, "ICU Physician's Role in Distributing Scarce Resources."
4. Roth, Loren H.; Meisel, Alan; and Lidz, Charles W. "Tests of Competency to Consent to Treatment." *American Journal of Psychiatry* 134 (1977): 279–84.
5. *Superintendent of Belchertown* v. *Saikewicz*, 370 N.E.2d 417 (Mass. 1977).
6. Annas, George J. "The Case of Mary Hier: When Substituted Judgment Becomes Slight of Hand." *Hastings Center Report* 14 (1984): 23–25.

7. U.S. Department of Army. "Do-Not-Resuscitate or 'No Code' Orders." Update Army Regulation 40-3, Chapter 19. February 15, 1985.
8. Sullivan, Ronald. "Hospital's Data Faulted in Care of Terminally Ill." *New York Times*, March 21, 1984, B1, B6.
9. American Heart Association and the National Academy of Sciences–National Research Council. "Standards and Guidelines for Cardiopulmonary Resuscitation (CPR) and Emergency Cardiac Care (ECC)." *Journal of the American Medical Association* 244 (1980): 453–509.
10. Uhlmann, Richard F.; Cassel, Christine K.; and McDonald, Walter J. "Some Treatment-Withholding Implications of No-Code Orders in an Academic Hospital." *Critical Care Medicine* 12 (1984): 879–81.
11. U.S. Department of Defense. "Policy on Identification, Surveillance and Disposition of Military Personnel Infected with HTLV III." Memorandum from the Secretary of Defense, October 24, 1985.
12. Smith, Paul. "Navy Forces Out Victims Who Admit Homosexual Contact." *Navy Times*, August 26, 1985, 4.
13. U.S. Department of Army, "Do-Not-Resuscitate or 'No Code' Orders."
14. U.S. Department of Army. "Withdrawal of Life Support." Letter from the Office of the Adjutant General to the Commanders of the Major Military Commands. August 30, 1985. Reference AR 40-3, Chapter 19.
15. Davis, Hal. "Hospital Sued for 20 M for Grandma's 'Deliberate Death.'" *New York Post*, June 6, 1984.

9

Mrs. Moore and the Doctor of Philosophy

Albert R. Jonsen

All ethics consultants have collections of cases in their memories and in their files. The cases serve as touchstones when we face new clinical situations, as examples when we teach and explain ethical issues, as reminders of what we have done well or poorly. This chapter draws on a case in my collection that poses some questions about the kind of work we do as ethics consultants. Each consultant probably has a similar case; mine has no claim to uniqueness. My purpose is to raise, in a concrete way, some key questions about ethics consultation to provoke wider discussion in the literature.

THE CASE

I was visiting a small community hospital in which our medical school maintains several clerkships and residency programs. Most of the medical students and residents had been my students at one time or another. I had given medical grand rounds in the morning and was passing the afternoon in the outpatient department. At about three o'clock, I was paged and, when I picked up the phone, the caller said, "We have an ethical emergency in the ER. Could you come over?"

When I arrived, I found a group of residents, medical students, and nurses. Behind a half-pulled curtain, an elderly woman, sitting up on a gurney, was being obstreperous. The intern told me that Mrs. Moore's left foot was gangrenous. Her landlady had called the police and asked them to take her to the hospital. She resisted and was removed bodily. The surgeon saw her immediately and told her the foot would have to be amputated. She refused and told him and all of the other personnel to get out; she had been screaming that she wanted to go home. She seemed to be in her eighties and apparently had no relatives. No one had been in touch with her landlady. The medical student who had tried to take her history then added, "Her foot is really a mess. It's covered with some kind of plaster. She said God had told her to cure her foot by putting plant food on it." I asked a few questions to ascertain the state of affairs, then said I would like to talk with Mrs. Moore.

I went behind the curtain. She had quieted down, but as soon as I entered she ordered me out in no uncertain terms. I ignored her request and said, "I'm Dr. Jonsen from the medical school." She asked me, "What kind of doctor are you?" I answered, "A doctor of philosophy." She responded tartly, "Well, then, what's your philosophy?" After that introduction, we were able to carry on a conversation. She quieted down, and spoke to me in a clear and coherent way. She was 87 years old and had lived alone in a trailer camp for the last 20 years. A month ago, her foot began to hurt. Her doctor came (she now gave his name and one of the medical students standing outside put in a call). The doctor had arranged for a visiting health aid. The woman was a thief, and Mrs. Moore had dismissed her two weeks before. Her foot had gotten worse, and about a week before our meeting, she said she had awakened with the "God-given inspiration" that applications of calcium might help. She had some plant food with bone meal in it and made a plaster. She thought it was getting better. She did not want to be in the hospital. When that doctor had told her that he was going to cut off her foot, she had refused. She knew she might die, but that was all right. She was 87 years old; she would not live long anyway. She did not want to lose her foot or her leg just to stay alive as a cripple for a year or so. In fact, she had been thinking about dying for several months. She had called her lawyer (whose name she gave in response to my question) and had a new will prepared. She had a little money and, since all her relatives were dead, she was giving most of it to the Lighthouse for the Blind. Her sister had been blind for the last 20 years of her life. The rest would go to the Presbyterian seminary.

That was Mrs. Moore's story. She told it in an eminently rational way, with the vocabulary and phrasing of an intelligent and educated woman. She was clearly oriented to person, place, and time and seemed quite aware of the nature of her problem and the consequences of her refusal. She concluded by asking if I would help to get her out of there and back to her home. As I left the cubicle, she called, "And find out who's going to pay for this. I didn't ask to come here and I won't pay anything." The ER staff had heard all of the conversation. We sat down to talk about Mrs. Moore.

All agreed, on the basis of what they had overheard, that Mrs. Moore was competent. The medical student readily confessed that Mrs. Moore had said "God-given inspiration," not "God told me," and acknowledged that the idea of a calcium cure was not irrational even if it was not scientific. They had little difficulty in seeing that Mrs. Moore was making a competent refusal of care and that they ought to respect that refusal. I briefly rehearsed the Mary Northern case from Tennessee and several of our California precedents. The resident then said, "Well, our real problem is how to make her comfortable and get her back home." She said that she would contact social services right away. At that moment, a call from the administrator came. I heard the resident say, "It would be a moral insult to submit that lady to a psychiatric examination. She's as sane as you or I." The group broke up as the resident went back to tell Mrs. Moore that they would just clean up her foot, put fresh bandages on it, and have her taken home.

DISCUSSION

That, then, is the case of Mrs. Moore and the doctor of philosophy. It raises a number of questions that are relevant to the definition of the work of an ethics consultant.

First, what was ethical about that consultation? We call ourselves ethical consultants. I was called to an "ethical emergency." I have always understood ethics to be a branch of moral philosophy. I was, in this instance, Mrs. Moore's doctor of philosophy. Yet, did I do or say anything particularly characteristic of moral philosophy? In a sense, I suppose I did. When Mrs. Moore asked, "What's your philosophy?", I could have responded with one of two statements — either "It is my philosophy that nothing should be done to you that is not for your good," or "Nothing should be done that is contrary to your competent wishes." In fact, I did answer with the second statement or something like it. In so doing, I had said something philosophical; I had expressed my belief in the moral primacy of personal autonomy. However, when we attend the occasional meeting of philosophers or read the *Journal of Medicine and Philosophy*, we recognize that the ethics of personal autonomy and the ethics of beneficence are conceptually complex. We are aware that it is not an easy matter to justify one or the other or, for that matter, to define the terms. Obviously, Mrs. Moore was in no mood to listen to a disquisition on the subject. Just as obviously, the staff was not ready to attend my lecture on Kant and Mill. Through a rather tortuous path, through many distinctions and qualifications, I had personally reached a conclusion about the ethical problem in Mrs. Moore's case, but I did not expose others either to my reasons or to the various problems that remain unresolved. Had I, then, performed an *ethical* consultation? What would Socrates have done? Are we merely the computerized version of the sage, providing conclusions out of our efficient but concealed program?

Second, what was the legal status of my intervention in the case? I assume that the legality would rest on some sort of license or recognized competence to do what I did. I have no license, except a certificate to perform cardiopulmonary resuscitation. As for my competence, whatever it is, it certainly is not in any way a trained and certified competence to perform any proper medical and health care activity other than cardiopulmonary resuscitation. Yet I carried out the equivalent of a mental status examination, on the basis of which Mrs. Moore was assessed as competent. I discussed the case, not in abstract terms, but with sufficient concreteness that certain decisions were made about her medical care. The consequences of those decisions were serious: Mrs. Moore died two weeks later, the result of sepsis that could have been prevented by surgical intervention. Thus, my role in the case was very much more like a medical consultant than an ethical consultant. Should I not bear the same responsibilities, be liable to the same sanctions?

Third, should I have intervened at all? Certainly, I was right to respond to the request but, on arrival, should I have listened to the staff's explanation of the problem, discussed the principal ethical and legal issues, and left? I am a teacher; my academic appointment designates me as a nonclinical professor. Should I not, then, limit my participation in such a case to a discussion with the staff and the students, leaving them to carry out all interactions with patient and family, assiduously avoiding all influence on their decisions that is not purely intellectual or informational? In this case and in many others, I see the patient or the family. Do we step beyond the limits of our charge? Should we view ourselves, and encourage others to view us, as clinicians as well as teachers?

Fourth, where does my consultation fit into the standard of care? In this case, my participation was accidental. It was a small hospital; many of the house officers and medical students and some of the attendants knew me and my work. I had given a lecture on medical ethics that morning, which most of them had attended. I had high visibility at that place and time. It was quite natural to call the ethicist. Had I been back at the medical school, with its five hospitals and myriad, mobile staff, my being summoned would have been equally accidental. On some services, I am known better than on others; some attending physicians frequently invite me, others never. Often, the summons comes after the case has become so confused and distressing that calling a neutral party is a last desperate step. Ethics consultation is certainly not considered an essential element in the care of the patient. (Indeed, it is often more directed to the care of the staff.) Yet all of us know of cases in which genuine ethical injury—the violation of rights and disrespect of personal dignity—has taken place, not because the staff was vicious but because they did not understand or appreciate the ethical dimensions of the case. Similarly, if the ethical problem lies at the heart of a decision, as it does in those agonizing moments when withholding or withdrawing care is being considered, should not consultation be more than accidental or occasional? Is ethical care a measure of the standard of care? Should ethics consultation be mandatory in certain kinds of cases, highly advisable in many others? Should the standards of the Joint Commission on Accreditation of Healthcare Organizations require a protocol for ethics consultations and evidence that they duly take place?

Mrs. Moore's case raises these four questions: What is an ethics consultation? What is the legal status of our consulting activity? Are we or should we be clinicians? How does our work fit into the quality of care provided to patients in our institutions? Doubtless, there are other questions raised by this case and many others. As ethics consultants, we need to produce for ourselves and for those with whom we work a clearer picture of our presence in the world of medicine and health care.

Part IV

Legal Implications and Standards

INTRODUCTION

Do physicians have a legal duty to seek ethics consultation? Do ethics consultants have a legal duty to inform the patient that they have been called in to help? What are the legal liabilities, if any, that ethics consultants or their institutions face? Part IV contains an essay on these legal questions by John A. Robertson, a scholar in law who is familiar with the clinical setting. No suits for "ethics malpractice" have, to our knowledge, been lodged against ethics consultants, although a hospital ethics committee has been named in one suit (*Bouvia* v. *High Desert Hospital*). Robertson's chapter is the first of such essays in the literature. He examines the scope and grounds of legal duties and privileges of ethics consultants and of the physicians who request their services.

What standards should be used for the evaluation of the services of ethics consultants? John C. Fletcher's chapter discusses the distinction between "formative" and "summative" evaluation. He outlines some basic steps by which institutions can evaluate their ethics consultation services, whether provided by an individual or a committee.

10

Clinical Medical Ethics and the Law: The Rights and Duties of Ethics Consultants

John A. Robertson

A significant development in the health care system in the last ten to fifteen years has been the emergence of medical ethics as an integral part of medical education and medical care. Revelations about excesses in human experimentation, the emergence of life-prolonging technologies (such as heart and kidney transplants, respirators, and dialysis), and the rising consumerism of the 1960s made physicians and the public aware that much of medical practice involves nonmedical ethical, legal, and social questions beyond the expertise of medicine itself.

One response to this awareness has been exogenous regulation of medical decisions by publicly articulated legal rules and norms, such as the Department of Health and Human Services rules for human experimentation, laws about brain death, informed consent, and the like. The power and authority, indeed the legitimacy, of medical hegemony has been questioned and directly confronted by substituting public norms for the nonmedical aspects of medical practice. The tension here is between public and professional control, with an ever-shifting balance among those elements.

A second development has been endogenous; that is, the incorporation of ethical training and awareness into medical education and training. The assumption here is that if doctors face and make ethical decisions, they should have training in such matters. This response has led to the development of courses in ethics, law, and related aspects of medical care in almost every medical school in the United States and the employment of philosophers, theologians, lawyers, and humanists by medical schools. It has also led, as part of this teaching role, to the increasing involvement of philosophers, lawyers, and ethicists in clinical medicine, as consultants and advisors to physicians, through attendance at the bedside, during teaching rounds, and on institutional review boards (IRBs). A closely related development has been the rise of in-house hospital ethics committees that may be consulted by physicians on a mandatory or optional basis as ethical problems arise, usually in the care and treatment of critically ill or dying patients.

We see, in short, the development of a new clinical role, an addition to the health care team that, in some cases, may be as important as its medical members. While the reasons for the emergence of the role are understandable, its scope and institutional posture are less clear. The rights and duties of ethics consultants are also unclear. This chapter will discuss the legal aspects of clinical medical ethics and medical ethics consultants, looking first at the physician's right and duty to consult or utilize the services of an ethics consultant and then turning to the legal rights and duties of the consultants. The goal is to produce a preliminary mapping in order to clarify and define the institutional parameters of the ethics consultant's role.[1]

THE PHYSICIAN AND THE MEDICAL ETHICS CONSULTANT

At the present time, medical ethics consultants function largely as adjuncts or assistants to physicians, either as individual consultants or as members of institutional committees that physicians choose to consult on an advisory basis. (On rare occasions, individual patients or families may consult an ethicist for help with a medical care decision.) Though not invariably so, ethics consultants become clinically involved only with the consent or request of the physician. This situation raises two issues: (1) the physician's legal right to call in a consultant, and (2) the physician's legal duty to do so.

THE PHYSICIAN'S RIGHT TO USE AN ETHICS CONSULTANT

In this context, "right" refers to the freedom to use an ethics consultant rather than the claim right on others to provide one.[2] The issue is whether consulting an ethicist or institutional ethics committee violates any legal or ethical duty the physician has to the patient. Two possible issues arise. One involves the broad area of confidentiality and concerns the physician's right to discuss a patient's case with another without the patient's consent; that is, must the physician ask the patient's permission to seek an ethics consultation? Must the patient be informed if the physician does consult an ethicist?

The physician probably does not have an obligation to consult the patient. Confidentiality is an important value in medicine, but it has never functioned to prevent physicians from seeking advice or consultation from others who may assist or improve the physician's handling of a particular case. Indeed, the patient is deemed to give implied consent to the physician seeking advice from others who are reasonably likely to help in management of the case. As Mark Siegler has shown, in a case of routine surgery, as many as 75 people may, as members of the total health care team, have legitimate access to a patient's medical records on the basis of implied consent.[3] A physician who discusses a case with an ethicist or a hospital ethics committee presumably would be acting for the patient's best interests as part of the care of the patient and would be privileged to do so as a matter of implied consent, unless the patient had given an explicit order to the contrary. Indeed, the law would not even require that the patient be informed that others had been consulted or had access to his or her records.

Bringing the consultant to the bedside is another matter. Here the relationship of the ethicist to the patient should be handled similarly to the relations between other consultants or students and the patient. Whether we view the doctor-patient relationship as a partnership, with the patient informed and consenting to all transactions, or a more paternalistic physician-guided model, simple courtesy and respect require that any consultant be introduced to the patient or patient's family and remain only with their permission. If, as is often the case, prevailing practice or custom does not generally call for the patient to be informed about the use or presence of a consultant, there would appear to be no reason why the ethicist should be treated differently. In either case, the physician might be discourteous.[4]

The question of a physician's right to resort to an ethics consultant raises the issue of the physician's discretion in management of a case. The patient's role in agreeing to or even being informed of the situation is secondary, even though consent to procedures or decisions made as a result of the consultation may be required. The relationship between ethicist and physician demands great respect for physician discretion in management of a case. The physician is consulting an ethicist for advice, clarification, and analysis of the ethical issues involved, but is not transferring decisional authority to the ethicist. As with other consultants, the ultimate decision about management of the case rests with the physician (and the patient), although it is made in light of the clarification and analysis of the consultant.

Given the nature of the arrangement between physician and ethicist-consultant, a physician would have no legal duty to take any particular action as a result of the ethics consultation. The physician's obligation to the patient continues to be to possess and use that degree of skill and care possessed and used by reasonable physicians in the same circumstances. While this duty may require seeking an ethics consultation and considering the advice proffered,[5] it requires the physician to act only as a reasonable physician would act in light of the information received. Thus, unless the decision is totally removed from the physician, there is no duty to follow the ethicist's advice or recommendation, though there is a duty to act reasonably in light of it. An ethics consultation will prevent a physician from claiming ignorance of the moral gravity of a situation, but the consultation alone will not mandate that the physician take any particular action.

THE PHYSICIAN'S DUTY TO OBTAIN AN ETHICS CONSULTATION

While the physician may be free to consult an ethicist without violating any duty to the patient, a major issue is whether the physician has a duty to do so. Physicians use consultants all the time. A central principle of medical ethics is that a physician seek a consultation when management of a case indicates the need for one. The law imposes this duty as well and will award damages to patients who have been injured by a physician's failure to seek a consultation in situations where other reasonable physicians would have obtained the advice of a consultant.

Does the physician's legal and ethical obligation to call in a consultant extend to an ethics consultant? There is a plausible case that it does in at least two circumstances. The first, and least controversial, is that there is such a duty when the hospital or institution explicitly imposes it, as it does with research with human subjects and sometimes with termination of treatment of the critically ill. In that case, failing to refer a case to an IRB or other ethics committee would violate an institutional and, in some cases, a state-imposed rule and could lead to damages on the basis of a negligence per se rule.

At the present time, with the exception of human subjects committees (IRBs), most institutions do not require ethics review or consultation. A survey of the President's Commission for the Study of Ethical Problems in Medicine found that only 17 of 400 hospitals with more than 200 beds had ethics committees, with 7 of these in New Jersey where we would expect such committees to have been formed as a result of the guidelines formulated in the Quinlan case.

A major issue relating to the use of ethics consultants thus concerns the extent to which hospitals and institutions should create ethics committees and then require that they be used in certain cases. This issue actually depends on a preliminary judgment that ethics committees are needed to prevent erroneous or inappropriate decisions in certain circumstances. Questions to be addressed concern defining the categories of cases that warrant review, designing a review process that will enhance accuracy without undue cost, and deciding whether review should be mandatory or optional for the physician and, in either case, whether the ethics committee's decision is merely advisory or must then be followed by the physician. While ethics committees are not yet well developed or widely used (other than in human experimentation), they have generated widespread interest, and it is likely that they will be further developed and expanded in the near future.

More controversial is the question of a duty to seek an ethics consultation when no hospital or institutional rule specifically requires it. The question of such a duty would arise, of course, only if an ethics committee were available on the premises. A legal duty to seek an ethics consultation would exist if a physician could be ordered to pay damages to a patient for failure to have obtained a consultation. The question is one of negligence: Is the failure to seek an ethics consultation in certain cases a matter of professional malpractice? To find a doctor liable for not seeking an ethics consultation, and thus the subject of a legal duty to do so, would depend on (1) the difference or impact an ethics consultant would have made in the handling of the case, and (2) the custom or practice of other physicians or the reasonableness of calling for an ethical consultation.

Under existing principles of malpractice law, damages could be awarded for the physician's failure to seek an ethics consultation only if the consultation would have improved the handling of a case. It seems clear that an ethicist or ethics committee could improve the handling of a case in many situations. While a physician may have had some college or medical school exposure to ethical issues, physicians will not always be adept at seeing ethical issues and problems. The extent to which issues of autonomy, beneficence, and justice arise in a case may not always be obvious, much less how conflicts among them should be resolved. Consider for a moment the complex ethical issues that arise in typical cases such as whether an elderly woman with a gangrenous leg may refuse amputation, whether physicians should acquiesce to parental wishes against surgery for a newborn with Down's syndrome, and whether intravenous feeding can be discontinued for a comatose patient.

Consultation with an ethicist or ethics committee may improve a physician's decisions in these cases, if only in clarifying the issues and conflicts and making the physician aware of the availability of materials concerning the ethical, legal, and policy aspects of such decisions. In many cases, the consultation could lead the physician to make decisions that are more respectful of patients' rights or interests than those that would have been made without the consultation (e.g., showing how the Down's syndrome child has rights to treatment that should be given priority over the parents' wishes, or that intravenous feeding may legally and ethically be stopped as the family wishes, even though the physician would wish to continue them).

Although the physician's recourse to an ethics consultation might help patients, there would be no legal duty to use this resource unless the applicable standard of care for patients in those circumstances would require the consultation. Under malpractice law, physicians are liable for omissions only if (1) the action would have benefited the patient (e.g., averted a harm) and (2) reasonable physicians in the same or similar circumstances would have performed the action. Therefore, for the physician to be considered liable and hence have a legal duty to seek an ethics consultation, a plaintiff claiming that the physician's choice to ignore ethical issues led to injury would have to show both that an ethics consultation would have prevented the injury and that other reasonable physicians in those circumstances would have sought a consultation. This standard depends in large part on the custom and practice of physicians. If a majority of physicians in those circumstances would have recognized that there were nonmedical ethical issues beyond their competence and sought an ethics consultation, there would be a much stronger case that the physician had a duty to consult an ethicist (although the respectable minority rule would still provide a defense in many jurisdictions).

But a majority of physicians do not now seek ethical consultations, and so no custom to that effect exists. However, it may still be possible to show or establish that a reasonable physician in those circumstances would call for a consultation rather than acting on his own. With all of the attention given to medical ethics and the increasing application of public or societal norms to medical practice, a reasonable physician should know that in certain areas (e.g., treatment issues pertaining to defective newborns, fetuses, the comatose, refusal of treatment, and experimentation), there are ethical questions that are beyond the physician's expertise and about which the public and law may have standards. Such questions, therefore, should not be handled by the physician without, at the very least, consulting in-house specialists on the subject.

A court holding that a physician has a duty to seek an ethics consultation, even though this is not yet a custom among a majority of physicians, would be setting a standard beyond medical practice. While such decisions by courts usually engender protest and controversy about unjustified and inexpert interference with the practice of medicine (see, for example, reactions to statute that tried to overrule *Helling* v. *Carey* and *Canterbury* v. *Spence*), the question is whether such a requirement can be justified in its own right. It is unlikely that a court will so rule, but it is possible and there is no reason why they should not. Requiring the physician, who is making a decision that may cause a patient's death, to examine the ethical issues involved in this decision with an expert on the ethics of such actions seems like a reasonable policy.

A further problem with maintaining a successful malpractice suit against a physician for failure to consult an ethicist concerns whether such a suit would lie in its own right or whether it would bolster a suit on other grounds (that is, in most cases the suit will claim that the physician was negligent in handling the case for some reason other than failure to seek an ethics consultation). However, making a decision on an ethical matter without expert advice could be evidence of negligence or recklessness. A physician who turned off a respirator or stopped feeding would be liable, because those actions violated a duty to the patient, whether or not an ethicist was consulted. If the physician claimed that he or she had acted reasonably in good faith, it would be harder to sustain that defense if an ethicist had not been consulted in a situation where reasonable physicians would recognize that a serious ethical problem existed.

THE LEGAL DUTIES OF THE ETHICS CONSULTANT

THE RIGHT TO GIVE ETHICAL ADVICE: LICENSING

Doctors, nurses, lawyers, and other professionals must be licensed to practice their professions. Ethics consultants give advice and make recommendations that can affect the lives of doctors and patients in significant ways. Must they be licensed as well? At the present time, the medical licensing acts do not cover the kinds of advice and services that medical ethicists provide. A common definition of the practice of medicine is "suggesting, recommending, prescribing or administrating any form of treatment, operation or healing for the intended palliation, relief or cure of any physical or mental disease, ailment, injury, condition or defect of any person."[6] An ethics consultant could attempt to practice medicine, but he or she could not both act as a consultant (e.g., in Terrence Ackerman's terms, "facilitating moral inquiry"[7]) and practice medicine within the meaning of the medical practice acts. Whether ethical consultants should be licensed in their own right will depend on future developments in the field.[8]

THE DUTY TO GIVE COMPETENT ADVICE

No cases involving ethics consultants have arisen, so the following comments about legal duties are based on analogies or generalizations about the legal duties that persons, particularly professionals, have when they undertake to perform certain tasks. Although malpractice suits against ethicists are so unlikely as to appear fancified, it is still useful to determine which legal duties might apply in order to better define the obligations of the ethics consultant's role.

The ethics consultant, like any other person who undertakes to act, advise, or provide services that could affect the lives or well-being of others in significant ways, could be held legally responsible for a failure to use due care and act reasonably in the consultant role. Such a question could arise in a suit brought by a patient or a physician who claimed to have been injured by the ethics consultant's actions. To win such a suit, the physician or patient would have to establish (1) that an ethics consultant had a duty to meet certain standards in his advice, (2) that the consultant failed to do so, and (3) that the failure caused the plaintiff's injury.

Establishing the ethics consultant's standard of care would be a central issue. As with physicians, the duty of care would depend upon what other reasonable ethicists would do in those circumstances, which would in turn be a function of the precise facts and situation. At a minimum, the ethicist would have to have a reasonable level of competency in describing, clarifying, and facilitating ethical analysis of a case, and then not overstep the bounds of analysis and clarification into normative ethics or substantive decision making in its own right. In short, the duty is to be a good, competent, reasonably humble ethicist. The malpractice would be in performing poorly in that role (e.g., omitting or misinforming about a key ethical issue, so that a major aspect of the case was missed, or preempting the decision by telling the physician what to do).

After establishing that the ethicist deviated in some significant way from good ethical or consultant practice in those circumstances, the plaintiff would then have to establish that the dereliction caused an injury. In a suit by a patient or a patient's family, the claim would be that the ethicist's advice or failure to give advice led, for example, to the patient being maintained for several extra days on a respirator. In a suit by a physician, the doctor would have to show that he or she had not merely made an unwise or unethical choice as a result of the ethicist's advice but had been injured as a result of the ethicist's advice. The clearest case of injury would be if the doctor made a decision, based on the ethicist's advice, that led to criminal, civil, or disciplinary action, and hence damages against the doctor. In either case, damages theoretically would lie against the ethicist, though suits are highly unlikely, if only because the damages may not be large enough to support a tort action. Indeed, the most likely suit against an ethicist would arise if a patient were suing a doctor and a hospital and added other parties and consultants, including the ethicist, as defendants.

The theoretical possibility of suit does highlight the need for ethicists to use due care in giving advice and not to overstep their bounds (as well as to arrange for insurance coverage by the institution). Ethicists can give bad or wrong advice, just as any consultant can. They can be arrogant, as if they think that they know the correct answer and insist that their advice be followed, or believe that they have an ethical duty to achieve certain goals and thus arrogate certain decisions to themselves. While such types may be rare and may not last long as ethics consultants, we must remember that ethicists too may act improperly.

To take but one example of consultant negligence (though not one arising in a clinical setting), consider the role that a priest-consultant played in the Phillip Becker case, in which the parents of a 12-year-old child with Down's syndrome opposed treatment of a ventriculo-septal defect and were upheld by the courts. Most commentators have been critical of the parents' decision and the court's finding because Phillip appeared likely to benefit from this surgery, and his parents did not appear to be acting for his best interests. It turns out that the parents' decision was based in part on advice received from a priest whom they had consulted about this case. It is not known whether the priest was trained in medical ethics or what reasoning he used. At the hearing before the court, the Beckers stated that their consultation with the priest led them to firmly oppose treatment that the doctors thought would extend their retarded son's life and prevent his suffering. A more accurate ethical analysis might have led to the opposite conclusion. While a suit against the consultant in this case may not have been appropriate, since causation would be difficult to prove, one can imagine similar situations in which a physician relies on an ethicist and makes decisions that hurt the patient and the physician.

THE ETHICS CONSULTANT AS WHISTLE BLOWER

Perhaps the most difficult issue in determining the ethicist's duties concerns situations where the ethicist learns of or sees a wrong done to a patient. As Terrence Ackerman shows in Chapter 2, the main function of the ethics consultant is "facilitating independent moral investigation by health professionals." The role is not to be a moral police officer, who identifies instances of clearly immoral behavior by health professionals; a patient advocate, whose primary duty is to protect the interests of patients; or a secular member of the clergy, whose duty is to inspire people to engage in morally appropriate behavior.

While this account of the ethicist's role is analytically sound, the question remains as to what the ethicist-consultant should do if he or she thinks a morally inappropriate course of action is taken in a case. Indeed, this issue is one with which ethicists are familiar because the question of duty to report wrong, or whistle blowing, is a common situation that ethicists discuss during their training.

The ethicist, of course, is in a similar bind. At some point, the duty to report wrongdoing may even cause the ethicist to risk his or her job. Two obligations must be distinguished: one is the specific duty toward a particular patient, and the other is the general duty to be concerned about institutional practices.

DUTY TO THE PATIENT

The issue here is whether an ethicist who is called in by a doctor as a consultant in a particular case has a duty to protect the patient when the doctor, despite the consultation, chooses a course of action that, in the ethicist's view, harms the patient.[9] Taking the repair of duodenal atresia in an otherwise healthy Down's syndrome child as an example, what should the ethicist do if the doctor, after hearing the ethicist's analysis of the child's rights, chooses to accept the parents' refusal to consent to surgery and orders that the child not be nourished?

Does the ethicist, because of his or her involvement as consultant, take on a duty to act for the well-being of the patient that did not exist before the consultation? Is the ethicist's duty merely to give a competent ethical analysis that will facilitate the physician's process of moral inquiry? If the ethicist's role is simply to facilitate moral inquiry, it would seem that it involves no independent duty to protect the patient. This question is at the very heart of the ethics of consultation. The medical consultant is chosen by the physician, reports only to the physician, does not manage the case alone, and merely facilitates the physician's medical management of the case. Yet the courts would probably find that if the consultant was clearly aware of improper management that would harm the patient, it would be his or her duty to protect the patient. By agreeing to advise the physician about this case, he or she takes on a duty to act for the patient's best interests. This duty includes rendering reasonably competent advice as a consultant and, arguably, performing whatever other actions are necessary to protect the patient. Of course, the evidence of harm and the need for intervention would have to be clear and strong for the courts to recognize this additional duty.

If the medical consultant has such a duty, then it is difficult to see why the ethics consultant should be treated differently. Although the ethics consultant's role is to facilitate the physician's moral inquiry as the physician and other decision makers attempt to resolve ethical dilemmas, the role is performed to help fulfill the goals of the doctor-patient therapeutic relationship, which entails some measure of respect and concern for the interests of the patient. In terms of both ethics and law, entering into a consultant relationship involves the assumption of a duty to act to protect the patient when the ethicist becomes aware of a clear threat of significant harm. To determine the scope of this duty and when it arises, we would have to analyze specific situations. However, an ethics consultant who did nothing when a doctor acquiesced to the parents' decision to discontinue treatment could probably be found civilly and criminally liable for not fulfilling a duty to the child (as could any other member of the medical team).

DUTIES TO OTHER PATIENTS: WHISTLE BLOWING IN THE INSTITUTION

Consider a case in which the ethicist has not been consulted about a particular patient but has learned of an ethically dubious institutional practice that affects a patient or patients. Does the role of an ethicist involve a duty to act to protect other patients by calling unethical practices to the attention of the relevant actors or by reporting such practices to appropriate institutional or other authorities? Unlike the situation in which the ethicist has consulted with a physician about a particular case, the ethicist is under no ethical or legal obligation (beyond what is expected of any person) to monitor, report, or otherwise improve institutional ethical practices.

An ethicist may be more ethically sensitive and aware and hence more likely than other persons to identify unethical conduct or practices. Greater knowledge may lead to greater anguish, as the ethicist must struggle more often and intensely with unethical situations. It may even be appropriate for an institution (or institutional committee, such as an IRB) to look to the ethicist to identify unethical practices and bring them to the attention of institutional authorities, just as it might expect an institutional lawyer to mention legal problems. The ethicist would not act as the "moral police" so much as an ethics consultant to the institutional authorities, to help them design and run an ethically sound institution. But the role of house ethicist does not in itself create any greater duty to take action. A patient injured by an unethical institutional or physician practice, about which the ethicist was aware but did nothing, would still have a much weaker claim than the ethicist, whose reluctance to act or speak out would not result in legal culpability for the patient's injury.

If this analysis is correct, the ethicist has no greater legal duty as a whistle blower than other parties involved in the patient's care. Such duties may, of course, arise as a moral or legal matter for all persons aware of an unethical situation. Imposing a higher duty on the ethicist would not be justified by his or her expertise in ethical matters. It might also hinder the acceptance of and recourse to the ethicist by those who most need the consultant's services.

NOTES

1. The issues here are really a subset of those that relate to the ethical and legal responsibilities of medical consultants, with a special application because of the nonmedical nature of the ethics consultation. There is a long history of concern for the ethics or etiquette of medical consultancy, having roots to some extent in physicians' desire to keep consultants from stealing their patients. The law is not particularly well developed, so consent and malpractice principles are simply applied to this new area.

2. A physician, however, could argue that a well-equipped institution should have an ethics consultant available just as it does medical specialists and allied services essential to good care.

3. Mark Siegler, "Confidentiality: A Decrepit Concept," *New England Journal of Medicine* 307 (1982): 1518–21.

4. An ethicist who is aware that a physician has not followed such common courtesy will face a personal and professional moral dilemma about introducing himself or herself to the patient or suggesting a different practice to the physician. This raises a variation on the whistle-blowing issue that clinical ethicists frequently confront.

5. Indeed, since the role of the ethics consultant will usually be to clarify and describe rather than to recommend or decide (that is, to do descriptive or metaethics rather than normative ethics), a recommendation may overstep the ethicist's rightful role.

6. See, e.g., *Gates* v. *Jensen* 595 P2d 919 (Wash.) 1979. Ark. Stat. Ann. 72-604(1).

7. See Chapter 2.

8. The question of whether ethics consultants practice law may also arise, since they often discuss cases and indeed may be the only source of legal information available to the doctor involved. Nonlawyer consultants should be wary of assuming that they know

the law and can expertly advise physicians — there have been many mistakes of this sort.

9. The ethicist on the ethics committee may also face a dilemma regarding whistle blowing in a case about which his committee has been consulted. However, as one of a collective of consultants, his duty is different or less imperative than if he were a consultant to a physician in a particular case.

11

Standards for Evaluation of Ethics Consultation

John C. Fletcher

At this early stage of the practice of ethics consultation in health care, is it reasonable to explore standards by which to evaluate this activity? This chapter argues that evaluation can be useful if approached within strict limits, and it outlines an approach to evaluation as a basis for discussion.

The discipline of evaluation research is a complex enterprise. In a volume on practical evaluation, Patton refers to more than 40 types of evaluation.[1] He shows that different types of evaluation serve different purposes. A major conceptual distinction between two types of evaluation, formative and summative, was introduced by Scriven in the context of curricular and education innovations.[2] "Formative" evaluation aims to refine or improve a program or activity, which forces one to think about what is intrinsic about the entity being evaluated. For example, if a service of providing ethics consultation were newly introduced in a hospital, an evaluation would be appropriate if aimed at improving or refining the service to its optimal state.

"Summative" evaluation, on the other hand, aims to judge the merit or worth of the program or activity by determining its effects or outcomes. This type of evaluation assumes that a clear set of goals and objectives of the program or activity had been established from the outset, including some norms against which the outcomes could be measured. It is unlikely that any institution has yet developed the grounds for a summative evaluation, as it would be surprising to find a health care institution in which goals and objectives of this activity had been carefully defined from the outset.

Who would presume to claim to be an "expert" in ethics consultation, qualified to judge the merit of a particular approach to consultation? To judge merit, one would have to estimate the "intrinsic property" of the entity being evaluated.[3] One approach to evaluation of merit is to compare how an entity conforms to standards upon which a group of experts agrees, or to compare an entity to others within the same class. The temper among ethics consultants is that to venture down the road of "expertness" and strict standardization in ethics consultation is to go in the wrong direction. If such is the case, formative evaluation is the best approach from which to construct standards for evaluation.

In addition to the embryonic state of the art of ethics consultation, the diversity of disciplines from which biomedical ethicists come is a major reason to select the formative rather than the summative direction. We are a diverse group of biomedical ethicists coming to a new field, to use Margaret Mead's phrase, like "immigrants in time."[4] Mead used this phrase to describe the cultural experience of those socialized before World War II compared with the experience of those born after the war. Those born earlier found the culture of the 1960s a "new world" of values and affluence, consisting of such drastic change as to be analogous to immigrating from an "old world" nation to a new nation. However, the move was not geographical but cultural, a journey in time and values. Bioethics is, by analogy, comparable to a new reality in time. We have immigrated from various disciplines that, like nations, have their own languages, standards, customs, and professional obligations. As a discipline, bioethics has been difficult to define, although some progress has been made in outlining the range of problems and systematic approaches involved.[5] Bioethics probably has more characteristics of a "movement" than an academic discipline, although "ethics" and "applied ethics" are clearly capable of definition as disciplines.

Now another new speciality or activity has arisen within the scope of bioethics, the provision of ethics consultation. And as immigrants, if the analogy is acceptable, we have the problems that immigrants usually have in the first and second generations. They must relate to a new people and culture. They worry about breaking old ties and seek to reestablish the old ties in a new place.

However, it is not too early to outline the first attempts at formative evaluation, aimed at reflection on what is intrinsic to ethics consultation and at improving or refining the activity. A formative evaluation can only be conducted when an activity, called "ethics consultation," is underway. Someone has to need it and someone or some group has to be designated to provide it. How far along should an institution be in ethics consultation before an evaluation would be helpful? It seems that there should at least be an ongoing service to evaluate, a definition of the activity, a protocol for consultation, and (if possible) a statement of goals for the program that have been endorsed by those in authority.

What is ethics consultation? Ethics consultation is the provision, on request, of clarification of options and recommendations, in the context of an ethical problem that arises in patient care or research. Much more work needs to be done, and will be done, on the intrinsic properties of ethics consultation in health care. But rather than press more deeply into the content of a "good" consultation, let us attempt to clarify the *process* of ethics consultation. The question can be reframed: what is an ethics consultation? One must at least describe and delineate the activity in order to locate what is to be evaluated. A minimalist definition is as follows: An ethics consultation is a meeting, or series of meetings on a continuum from "informal" to "formal," between person(s) in need of help with an ethical problem and person(s) appointed to provide such help.

The concepts of informal and formal consultation were explored in a questionnaire given prior to the First National Conference on Ethics Consultation in 1985.[6] The results of the questionnaire showed that ethicists participate in about three times as many informal as formal consultations. As an example, an informal consultation occurs when Dr. X stops the bioethicist on the street outside the hospital and hurriedly raises a question, "By the way, should a normal volunteer in a family studies program of genetic disorders be told that his chromosomes were found to be XYY?" And then hē says that he is on his way to the Middle East and will return in a month.

Informal consultations often lead to more extended, formal consultations, which have many of the same characteristics as medical consultations. A formal consultation has at least these features:

1. A request for help with an ethical problem in a case or for information or interpretation of institutional policy that relates to a case;

2. A response by the consultant that may involve negotiation about (a) what is being requested by the consultant (i.e., clarification of options and recommendations), and (b) protection of the anonymity of the person who requests help;

3. An entry into the case by the consultant that may involve (a) seeing the patient at the request of the physician, (b) gathering facts about the question(s) under consideration, (c) interviewing others, (d) calling on other disciplines for assistance, (e) referral of aspects of the problem that are the responsibility of other disciplines, (f) clarification of options, and (g) recommendations;

4. The physician's or another health professional's note in the patient's chart that ethics consultation was obtained, and the consultant's note on the outcome of the consultation, recorded in the patient's chart or elsewhere;

5. A report of the consultation for the record, hospital ethics committee, or supervisor; and

6. A follow-up by the consultant with the principal parties in the consultation, if available, as to final outcome and evaluation of strengths and weaknesses of the service provided.

An early, formative evaluation could focus upon the important turning points in the evaluation process itself. The steps outlined below could be used as points for evaluation, while the questions raised in the outline could serve as data points in the evaluation.

POINTS FOR EVALUATION

1. Someone asks for help (Who? How directly?)
2. Consultant tests and negotiates (How clearly?)
   a. What is the ethical problem? (Referral?)
   b. What is being requested?
      • Clarification of options
      • Recommendations
3. Entry into the case (Timeliness? Clarity of role?)
   • Seeing patient at physician's request
   • Interviewing others in the case
   • Calling on other disciplines for assistance
   • Clarification of options
   • Recommendations by request
4. Patient's chart (Is it done? Helpful to others?)
   • Physician's note on request for ethics consultation
   • Ethics consultant's note
5. Report of consultation (Is it done? Used?)
6. Follow-up with principal parties (Is it done?)
   • Final outcome
   • Evaluation (strengths/weaknesses)

Some clarification of these turning points in the consultation process is indicated. First, someone asks for help, someone is unhappy, or someone has a problem; and that someone either telephones or stops you in the hall or comes up to you in the cafeteria or knocks on the door. Who is it? Who is requesting the consult? At the outset, the major issue is whether or not it is a direct request. Is this person speaking on her or his own behalf, or are they pointing to someone else who has a prob-

lem? Do they have a problem or are they bringing you someone else's problem? The consultant should be in touch with the
primary person who suffers the problem or who raised the
question; otherwise, one becomes "triangled" between a third
party and the primary party, who may or may not have an
ethical problem. We might ask ourselves how adept we are in
eliciting directness from the person who presents the problem
and how quickly we are able to be in touch with the person who
is most ethically troubled. Working this out in the beginning,
getting off on the right foot, can be a difficult lesson to learn,
especially when one has a desire to be helpful and to be
accepted in the institution.

Moving to the second step, the consultant tests the person
who presents the problem or, moving past the secondary car-
rier to the person or group most troubled, one begins to test
and negotiate about the problem itself. The test question is,
what is the *ethical* problem here? If there is really another type
of problem (e.g., legal, social, psychological, or unproductive
staff conflict), then a referral to another source is indicated.
Usually, some sorting out is needed to distinguish the ethical
dimension of a multifaceted problem from other dimensions.
Some useful questions to identify ethical problems are: Is
someone's (e.g., the patient's) welfare at stake? Are well-known
moral obligations in conflict? Are professional-ethical standards in conflict (e.g., between physicians and nurses)? Is a
policy of the institution with ethical content being questioned
or in need of clarification? Has a promise been broken or is it
in need of renegotiation? Is someone's right to raise an ethical
question being challenged?

Usually, the person would not be calling if there were not
an ethical problem. But it needs to be broken down and separated, and the parts of the problem that belong to other colleagues need to be referred. Otherwise, other colleagues in the
institution find out, much to their chagrin, that the ethics
consultant is working on their territory. Each of us knows how
it feels to learn that someone has been operating on our territory. If consultants frequently incur the anger of other professionals because they are functioning as psychiatrists, lawyers,

or physicians without the proper license, then an evaluation would reveal that faulty moves are being made in the crucial early stages of a consultation.

It is vital to meet face-to-face with the person who calls or presents the problem. The telephone is an extremely poor instrument through which to conduct a consultation, although consultations often begin on the telephone. If an ethics consultation entails a meeting or series of meetings, they should be arranged as soon as possible. Some consultations may be done by telephone when absolutely necessary, but such an arrangement is never optimal.

Assuming that an ethical problem exists that needs resolution, the next step is to determine what is being requested of the consultant. The question must be asked (followed by a statement to help the requester decide): "Doctor, what do you want from me? I agree with you that you have an ethical problem. I can provide help in two ways. I can help you and your colleagues and the patient clarify the options, and I can make a recommendation, but you must ask for it and so indicate in the record." Unless recommendations are requested, it may be easy to ignore them. If a consultant is formally asked for recommendations, these should be formally rendered.

It is sometimes necessary to negotiate about protecting the anonymity of the caller. Calls come in which, after discussion, appear to amount to whistle blowing. Protecting the well-being of whistle blowers, particularly in a large government research hospital, is an important task. Clients need to be reassured that they will not be punished for going to the ethics consultant, and the consultant must be backed up by the institution. However, it may not be possible to guarantee the person protection from authorities. If legal or regulatory problems are involved, one is at times obliged to reveal the source of the original report of a problem. Although the consultant may do everything possible to protect the client's reputation, security, and position in the institution, it is not always possible to keep the report itself a secret.

The third step is the entry into the case. An evaluation could focus on whether we make timely responses and entries into cases. Also, do we make the role of an ethics consultant clear as we are entering the case? Do we help other people to clarify and clear up role confusion? If a physician requests ethics consultation regarding a patient, then at the physician's request, the consultant should see the patient at the earliest possible time. If the patient is capable and conscious, she or he should be informed that the physician faces an ethical problem and has requested help from a consultant appointed by the institution for this purpose.

The consultant must be free to gather all the facts necessary and to interview, without interference, anyone in the institution who is related to the case. Next, the consultant should be free to call upon other disciplines for assistance. If very difficult emotional or family problems emerge in the case, or if serious conflict involving a history of poor morale or lack of interdisciplinary respect appears between staff, the consultant does not have the expertise to deal with the problem and must be able to call on a liaison-consultant in psychiatry or social work, or another source of help, to cope with the situation. Legal problems require the involvement of the hospital lawyer.

The clarification and recommendation of options, if requested, is the most important turning point from the standpoint of the ethical content of the consultation. One should work from sources that have high standing in the practice of medicine and research. Preparation for the meeting in which options will be explored with decision makers is a vital step. Some cases involve "ethics emergencies" in which views must be quickly explored and evaluated. However, normally there is time to prepare, and one should at least outline on a sheet of paper the options and major sources of guidance to back them up. If a recommendation has been requested, it should be delivered in writing if time permits. If the recommendations are delivered verbally, they should be accompanied with references to the literature, important positions of groups that have studied the question, or institutional policy statements. If a written recommendation is requested, the consultant might enter it in the patient's chart and give a copy to the physician, his or her supervisor, and the clinical director.

The next step is the patient's chart. Is a note by the ethics consultant entered, and is it helpful to others? Not everyone in a unit can be included in the meeting, and the patient's chart is not a place to write minutes of the meeting. Chart notes need to be clear and instructive to those who read them. (I always request that the physician note that an ethics consult was requested, and I enter my note at the appropriate page in the progress notes.)

The fifth step is the report of the consultation. But do we make reports? It is difficult and time consuming, but it is important to have a good form of reporting and to be able to see that the results are being used.

The final step is follow-up with the principal parties in the case, depending upon how the case evolved and who was involved. Some cases have only two people involved (a physician and patient) and some grow to casts of dozens. Follow-up involves two dimensions: Did people, especially other professionals, do what they said they would do? If referrals were made to psychiatrists, social workers, or a lawyer, what happened as a result? If your colleague has not told you the results, and your part in the case is over, a call is needed. Second, the consultant needs to learn the strengths and weaknesses of his or her approach and teaching in the case. The question needs to be asked, what was helpful or unhelpful?

Thorough discussion of the results of case consultation are linked to two ongoing institutional needs, education of staff in biomedical ethics and development of policy positions or statements. Bringing staff together for a retrospective review of a very controversial and interesting case provides a focus for more education than one can normally provide while doing the consultation. Also, consultation reveals the "soft spots" in institutional policy development where clearer guidance is needed. An existing policy statement might be challenged in an effective way during a consultation. When these needs arise, the task of strengthening the policy should be referred to the proper body.

We have focused on evaluating the process of ethics consultation. What about the content of the guidance or recommendations given? How adequate and sound is the guidance? How fairly and comprehensively are the options presented? Even in a formative evaluation, it is impossible to avoid issues of merit and worth. At a minimum, an institution must formulate goals for an activity or program which will form the basis of a more *substantive* evaluation of ethics consultation. If a program of ethics consultation is to be improved in process and content, what goals ought to be served to improve the effort?

Three important goals of ethics consultation are as follows:

1. To resolve ethical problems with optimal participation;

2. To reflect with decision makers on the major sources of ethical guidance for the problems at hand; and

3. To increase knowledge of ethics (i.e., knowledge of self, others, and the bodies of knowledge that comprise biomedical ethics).[7]

The first goal is to resolve ethical problems with optimal participation. If biomedical ethics is a social enterprise, rather than the province of experts, then optimal participation should be the norm. A convincing way to assure health care professionals that bioethicists do not intend to replace them in terms of clinical responsibility is to assure each person with a stake in the problem a share in the resolution of the problem. Everyone has a job to do and a unique contribution to make to the discussion and problem-solving efforts.

Second, major resources for ethical guidance (i.e., those representing the best thinking to date on the problem) should be used when reflecting with decision makers on the problem at hand. Criteria for selection of the best material include considerations based on good evidence, which conform to logical requirements, and the attempt to maintain continuity with major ethical traditions in the society. Whenever possible, it is helpful to provide copies of important articles in the literature, summaries of views, or outlines of the possible positions that might be taken on the problem. The recommendations and conclusions of the two national commissions on biomedical ethics in research and medicine are also helpful in providing resources and recommended guidance. Of course, if the institution has policy statements on the problem at hand, written copies should be made available to all concerned.

The third goal is to increase knowledge of ethics in general, as well as biomedical ethics. Biomedical ethics is a subset of general social ethics. One hardly ever has a chance to teach or communicate the large framework of social ethics in the context of case consultation. But one does have a chance in lectures, ceremonies, or other occasions when the time comes for traditions, symbols, and heritage to be displayed. Medical and nursing personnel need to be reminded that their professional ethics are derived from and accountable to larger systems.

Involvement in ethics consultation necessitates reflection on one's motivation, one's personality or character, and one's strengths and weaknesses, as well as on how one knows the others involved in the case, and how motivation and intent come into play in different persons. Self-knowledge and knowledge of others is one of the two main purposes of ethics, and the provision of guidance is the second. Neither of these goals is abstract. Respect for others presumes a capacity for and an interest in knowing them more deeply. To promote this kind of knowledge in the institution, as well as the special sources of guidance on biomedical ethics, is a goal with a practical outcome. A climate can be created in which persons become more open and capable of responding to significant ethical crises by virtue of their interest and experience in dealing with the smaller, more routine daily problems that may also be laden with ethical significance. Practice on the small problems leads to deeper resources for responses to the large ones.

NOTES

1. Michael Q. Patton, *Practical Evaluation* (Beverly Hills, CA: Sage Publications, 1982) 44–47.
2. Michael Scriven, *The Methodology of Evaluation*. Monograph Series in Curriculum Evaluation, No. 1 (Chicago: Rand-McNally, 1967).
3. Egon G. Guba and Yvonna S. Lincoln, *Effective Evaluation* (San Francisco: Jossey-Bass, 1981), 45.
4. Margaret Mead, *Culture and Commitment* (Garden City, NY: Natural History Press/Doubleday and Co., 1970), 72.
5. Warren T. Reich, *Encyclopedia of Bioethics*, 4 vols. (New York: Free Press, 1978).
6. The questionnaire and a summary of the results are included in the appendix of this book.
7. These goals were formulated at the National Institutes of Health (NIH) with the help of Maxwell Boverman, consultant to the NIH's bioethics program, and the liaison group, composed of 14 persons who assisted with the task of ethics consultation in the clinical center. The group was formed in the spring of 1985, after the medical board of the hospital stated that it did not desire an institutional ethics committee such as those established widely in other health care settings. As an alternative, a group was assembled to share the responsibility and to broaden the coverage for ethics consultation. This group was composed of seven physicians (including three psychiatrists, a neurologist, an oncologist, an internist, and a cardiologist) and seven other health care professionals (including two nurses, a social worker, a chaplain, a hospital lawyer, a genetic counselor, and a patient representative). Each was selected because of an interest in bioethics and the likelihood of being in an area of the hospital in which ethical problems frequently arise. The group met monthly for training in ethics consultation and to reflect on cases in which an ethics consultation was provided. Wherever possible, the persons directly involved in the case were invited to the case review.

Appendix

A Survey of Ethics Consultants

The questionnaire that follows was sent to each person who attended the First National Conference on Ethics Consultation in Health Care. Completion of the questionnaire was voluntary. However, each participant was asked to obtain a letter from the chief executive officer of the health care facility in which he or she gave consultation. The letter was to verify that ethics consultation was a recognized duty performed by the individual.

The questionnaire was developed by John C. Fletcher with the help of Gerald C. Macks, a management systems analyst in the Office of the Director, Clinical Center, NIH. The costs of administering the questionnaire and analyzing the answers were supported by a grant from the Eberhard Foundation (Exton, Pennsylvania). The instrument and discussion of findings from the responses of 38 (of 53) participants are included so that readers can appreciate the backgrounds, locations, and major variables in ethics consultation in this particular group.

Part I: Questionnaire

THE ETHICS CONSULTANT

A. Professional Background

1. Name: Last_____ First_____
    Middle initial_____
2. Age:_____
3. Please check if you have attached your CV_____
4. Please circle the graduate and professional degree(s) you
    have earned:

J.D.	M.D.	M.Div.
M.H.L.	M.S.W.	R.N.

    Ph.D. (In what discipline?_____)
    Other graduate or professional degrees that you hold?
    _____

B. The Ethics Consultant and the Institution

1. What is the title of your current position?
    Title:_____
    Institution:_____
    Location:_____
2. What was your last position before assuming your current
    position?
    Title:_____
    Institution:_____
    Location:_____
3. What institution employs you as an ethics consultant?
    Institution:_____
    Location:_____
4. For what else are you responsible in the institution in
    which you serve as ethics consultant?
    _____
    _____
    _____
    _____

5. What institution pays you?

   _____

6. Is part of your salary designated as compensation for ethics consultation?
   Yes_____ No_____

7. Who hired you?
   Name:_____
   Title:_____
   Institution:_____

8. In which department, service, or administrative branch is your position located?

   _____

9. How long have you been in your current position?
   _____Years _____Months

10. Who had the greatest influence in developing the position you now hold?
    Name:_____
    Title:_____
    Institution:_____

11. Do you have a written job or position description?
    Yes_____ No_____ If yes, please attach a copy.

12. Who is your administrative supervisor or superior?
    Name:_____
    Title:_____

13. To whom does he or she report?

    _____

14. Are your services as an ethics consultant described in hospital brochures, directories, or handbooks?
    Yes_____ No_____ If the answer is yes, to whom are your services made known? Please circle answer(s):
    Patients   Relatives   Medical Staff
    Hospital Staff   Students   Community

15. Does someone cover the ethics consultation service for you when you are away?

Yes_____ No_____ If yes, who?

_____

16. Do you regularly make rounds or make yourself otherwise visible in special areas of the hospital in which ethical problems frequently arise?
Yes_____ No_____ If yes, please circle the sites you visit most frequently:

Emergency Room	Intensive Care Unit	Neonatal ICU
OB-GYN	Oncology	Pediatrics
Psychiatric Unit	Research Units	Surgery

Other?_____

17. Does your institution have a Hospital Ethics Committee or its equivalent for ethical issues that arise in patient care?
Yes_____ No_____
If yes, what is the name of this group?

_____

18. Is your institution in the process of beginning a Hospital Ethics Committee?
Yes_____ No_____

19. If anwer to 17 is yes, do you serve on this group?
Yes_____ No_____ If yes, please circle role:
Chairman   Consultant   Member

20. How closely coordinated is the ethics consultation service in your institution with the committee named in question 17? Please circle the appropriate answer:
Closely   Related but independent
Loosely   Not at all related   Not relevant

21. How closely coordinated is the ethics consultation service in your institution with the work of hospital legal counsel? Please circle the appropriate answer:
Closely   Related but independent
Loosely   Not at all related   Not relevant

22. Does your institution have an Institutional Review Board or its equivalent for prior review of research?
Yes_____ No_____

23. If answer to 22 is yes, do you serve on this group?
Yes_____ No_____ If yes, please circle your role:
Chairman   Consultant   Member

CONSULTATION

1. Before you took your present position, did you have formal training in consultation?
Yes_____ No_____
If yes, please circle source of training:
Behavioral Sciences
Consultation-Liaison Psychiatry
Organizational Development
Other?_____

2. Have you occupied a previous position in which you offered consultation?
Yes_____ No_____ If yes, what position?

_____

3. If the answer to 2 is no, was your first experience in consultation "on the job"?
Yes_____ No_____

4. Did anyone help to educate or train you in the concepts and skills needed for consultation in your present position?
Yes_____ No_____

5. If the answer to 4 is yes, who helped you?

_____

What is his/her professional discipline?_____

The next few questions use a distinction between "formal" and "informal" case consultation. Strict lines are impossible to draw, but gradations of formality exist from the strictly formal to "curbstone consultation." A consultation that begins informally may also result in a formal consultation.

A formal consultation has at least these features:

1. A request for help with an ethical problem in a case or for information or interpretation of institutional policy that relates to a case;

2. A response by the consultant that may involve negotiation about (a) what is being requested of the consultant: i.e., clarification of options, recommendations, etc., (b) protection of the anonymity of the person who requests help, etc.;

3. An entry into the case by the consultant that may involve (a) seeing the patient at the request of the physician, (b) gathering facts about the question(s) under consideration, (c) interviewing others, (d) calling on other disciplines for assistance, (e) referral of aspects of the problem that are the responsibility of other disciplines, (f) clarification of options, and/or (g) recommendations;

4. The physician's or another health professional's note in the patient's chart that ethics consultation was obtained, and the consultant's note on the outcome of the consultation, recorded in the patient's chart or elsewhere;

5. A report of the consultation for the record, hospital ethics committee, or supervisor, etc.;

6. A follow-up by the consultant with the principal parties in the consultation, if available, as to final outcome and evaluation of strengths and weaknesses of the service provided.

An informal consultation may involve one or more features of formal consultations.

If you keep records of consultations, please answer questions 6, 7, and 8 with the precise number and write R (for Records) after the number; if you estimate the numbers, please write E (for Estimate) after the number:

6. How many formal case consultations did you provide in
   1980_____; 1981_____; 1982_____;
   1983_____; 1984_____?

7. How many informal case consultations did you provide in
   1980_____; 1981_____; 1982_____;
   1983_____; 1984_____?

8. How many consultations to interpret institutional policy in
   1980_____; 1981_____; 1982_____;
   1983_____; 1984_____?

9. Do you keep a written record of your consultations?
   Yes_____ No_____

10. If the answer to 9 is yes, do you regularly submit your
    written consultation reports to someone?
    Yes_____ No_____ If the answer is yes, to whom?

    _____

11. Has the question ever arisen as to whether your consulta-
    tion reports or written notes about the cases would be
    discoverable in a court of law?
    Yes_____ No_____

12. Do you purposely not write case consultation reports or
    keep notes for fear that these would be discoverable?
    Yes_____ No_____

13. In formal consultations, do you regularly write in the
    patient's chart?
    Yes_____ No_____ Only if requested_____

14. Do you have "jurisdiction" in specific issues in the sense
    that hospital staff are obliged to consult you on cases that
    involve these issues?
    Yes_____ No_____
    If yes, what are these issues?

    _____

    _____

15. If answer to 14 is yes, are hospital staff *obliged* to follow
    your advice in these cases?
    Yes _____ No_____

16. Does anyone consult with you about your consultations, i.e., provide a source of reflection, criticism, encouragement, support?

Yes_____ No_____ If yes, please answer:

Name:_____

Position:_____

Discipline:_____

17. Please review the list of 21 issues below. Which issues arise with the most frequency in your practice of ethics consultation? Please rate the frequency on a scale of 0–4. 0 = Never, 1 = Rarely, 2 = Occasionally, 3 = Often, 4 = Very frequently, X = No such unit or activity exists in my institution.

Issues	*Degree of Frequency*
A. Abortion choices	_____
B. Behavior problems in patients	_____
C. Brain death determinations	_____
D. Competence to consent to medical care	_____
E. Competence to consent to research	_____
F. Complaints about behavior of personnel	_____
G. Confidentiality	_____
H. Do-not-resuscitate orders	_____
I. Fetal research	_____
J. Full disclosure of diagnosis/prognosis	_____
K. Genetic counseling: directive/nondirective	_____
L. Iatrogenic events: full disclosure	_____
M. Macroallocation issues	_____
N. Microallocation issues	_____
O. Organ donor issues	_____
P. Refusal of treatment in nonterminal cases	_____
Q. Removal of life supports in terminal cases	_____
R. Research with children	_____
S. Research with mentally impaired subjects	_____
T. Selective nontreatment of high-risk newborns	_____
U. Sterilization	_____

Please add others not covered by list:

V._____   _____

W._____   _____

X._____   _____

Y._____   _____

Z._____   _____

18. Which of the 21 issues are least or most difficult for you as an *ethics* consultant? One measure of difficulty is that of achieving resolutions that are ethically consistent from case to case (i.e., we should treat similar cases similarly). Which issues cause you the most difficulty in terms of inconsistency of outcomes, and for which do you frequently need to search for justifiable "exceptions"? Please rate the degree of *ethical* difficulty according to a scale of 0–4. 0 = Never, 1 = Rarely, 2 = Occasionally, 3 = Often, 4 = Very frequently, X = No such unit or activity exists in my institution.

Issues	*Degree of Frequency*
A. Abortion choices	_____
B. Behavior problems in patients	_____
C. Brain death determinations	_____
D. Competence to consent to medical care	_____
E. Competence to consent to research	_____
F. Complaints about behavior of personnel	_____
G. Confidentiality	_____
H. Do-not-resuscitate orders	_____
I. Fetal research	_____
J. Full disclosure of diagnosis/prognosis	_____
K. Genetic counseling: directive/nondirective	_____
L. Iatrogenic events: full disclosure	_____
M. Macroallocation issues	_____
N. Microallocation issues	_____
O. Organ donor issues	_____
P. Refusal of treatment in nonterminal cases	_____
Q. Removal of life supports in terminal cases	_____
R. Research with children	_____
S. Research with mentally impaired subjects	_____
T. Selective nontreatment of high-risk newborns	_____
U. Sterilization	_____

Please add others not covered by list:

V._____   _____
W._____   _____
X._____   _____
Y._____   _____
Z._____   _____

19. Are you consulted by hospital administrators as a resource
    person on institutional policy interpretations? These
    requests may not necessarily relate to actual cases of
    patient care. Please circle your answer:
    Very frequently   Frequently   Occasionally
    Hardly ever   Never

COLLABORATION WITH OTHER DISCIPLINES

A collaborator is one who works jointly with you to facilitate
ethics consultation, often takes a role in cases, and provides
insight and assistance toward the resolution of the case.

1. Do you have other major collaborators in providing ethics
   consultation? Please circle your answer:
   More than one   One   One being prepared   No

2. Are your major collaborators also the main sources of
   referrals for your cases in ethics consultation? Or do your
   referrals come from other sources with greater, the same,
   or less frequency?

   In the first column, please indicate the discipline/specialty
of your major collaborator(s). If you have only one major collaborator, put 1 in the first column opposite his or her
discipline/specialty. If two or more, rank them 1, 2, 3, etc. in
terms of how closely you collaborate. In the second column,
rank the sources from which you most frequently receive referrals for ethics consultation. The most frequent source ranks as
1, the next as 2, etc.

Discipline	Major Collaborators	Sources of Referrals
A. Administrator	_____	_____
B. Cardiologist	_____	_____
C. Chaplain	_____	_____
D. Clinical Investigator	_____	_____
E. Endocrinologist	_____	_____
F. Genetic Counselor	_____	_____
G. Internist	_____	_____
H. Lawyer	_____	_____
I. Medical Geneticist	_____	_____
J. Neonatologist	_____	_____
K. Nephrologist	_____	_____
L. Neurologist	_____	_____
M. Nurse	_____	_____
N. Obstetrician-Gynecologist	_____	_____
O. Oncologist	_____	_____
P. Patient Representative	_____	_____
Q. Pediatrician	_____	_____
R. Philosopher	_____	_____
S. Psychiatrist	_____	_____
T. Psychologist	_____	_____
U. Social Worker	_____	_____

Other: Please add

V. _____	_____	_____
W. _____	_____	_____
X. _____	_____	_____
Y. _____	_____	_____
Z. _____	_____	_____

3. If your major collaborator is a psychiatrist, is he or she:
   a. In the Department of Psychiatry?
      Yes_____ No_____
   b. In the Liaison-Consultation Psychiatry Service?
      Yes_____ No_____
   c. From outside the institution?
      Yes_____ No_____

4. If your collaborator is a psychiatrist, who pays for this service?

   _____

5. What type of service is rendered by the psychiatrist?
    Please check the relevant answer(s):
    a. Direct service　　　　　　　　　　　　_____
    b. Examinations for competence　　　_____
    c. Diagnosis　　　　　　　　　　　　　_____
    d. Other (please describe):　　　　　_____

6. How often do you use the services of a psychiatrist in
    ethics consultation? Please circle your answer:
    Very frequently　　　Often　　　　　　Occasionally
    Rarely　　　　　　　　Never

7. If you use the services of a psychiatrist in ethics consulta-
    tion, how many contacts did you have in the past
    year?_____

8. If you use a psychiatrist to help with emotional problems
    attendant to providing ethics consultation, what are the
    problems that most need his or her attention? Please assign
    a rank to the frequency of the problem, on a scale of 0–4.
    0 = Never,　1 = Rarely,　2 = Occasionally,　3 = Often,
    4 = Very frequently.
    a. Communication problems:
       1. Between ethics consultant
          and physicians　　　　　　　　　_____
       2. Between ethics consultant
          and administration　　　　　　　_____
       3. Between physicians　　　　　　　_____
       4. Between nurses and physicians　_____
       5. Between patient and hospital staff　_____
       6. Between patient, family,
          and hospital staff　　　　　　　_____
       7. Between members of hospital
          ethics committee　　　　　　　　_____
    b. Emotional problems of patient　　_____
    c. Poor morale of hospital staff　　　_____
    d. Role clarification (of ethics consultant)　_____
    e. Support (emotional and intellectual,
       of the ethics consultant)　　　　　_____

f. Other problems (please describe):

_____

_____

9. If you use the services of another person besides a psychiatrist for such problems, in what discipline/specialty is he or she?

_____

10. How often do you use these services?
Frequently_____ Occasionally_____
Rarely_____

11. How many contacts did you have with this individual in the past year? _____

REMARKS OR COMMENTS

Please expand on anything you want to add, or please note anything that was overlooked.

PART II: SUMMARY OF FINDINGS

DESCRIPTIVE STATISTICS

Background

Thirty-eight ethics consultants participated in the survey. Their ages ranged from 33 to 58, with an average age of 43. Twenty held Ph.D.s. Other degrees were M.Div. (6), M.A. (5), M.D. (4), J.D. (3), R.N. (3), Other (6). Philosophy and theology/divinity were the most frequently represented disciplines among the respondents.

The sample was nearly evenly divided with respect to academic and nonacademic titles. Most participants held academic positions formerly, and half of those positions were in ethics. The majority of respondents were employed and paid by universities, hospitals, clinics, and medical centers. Employees of health care corporations were also represented. Primary responsibilities were listed as education or teaching, committee work, and research.

Most respondents held consulting positions in medically related departments such as medicine, nursing, or health care. The average respondent had been in his or her position about 5½ years. Two-thirds of the participants had held their positions between six months and 10½ years. Frequently named sources of influence in developing the respondents' positions were faculty members, the respondents themselves, or program directors. The majority of the sample worked in positions with written job descriptions and had their services described in brochures, directories, or handbooks. Their services were most often made known to colleagues on medical or hospital staffs. Deans, department chairs, mission directors, and program directors were most often named as respondents' supervisors. Less than half the sample reported that they had someone to cover the ethics service when they were away.

Despite the fact that many respondents were associated with medical institutions, very few reported that they made rounds. For those who did, intensive care, neonatal ICU, and pediatrics were visited most frequently. Only a minority, about one-third of the respondents, served on an ethics committee or equivalent group. Of those who were on such a committee, most were members, as opposed to consultants or chairpersons. Most of the survey participants said there was some degree of coordination or relationship between the ethics service and the committee on which they served. Most also reported some relationship between the ethics service and the hospital legal counsel. More than half were members of institutional review boards or the equivalent.

Consultation

Fifty percent of the sample had formal training in consultation, mostly in psychiatry and the behavioral sciences. Most respondents had some previous consultation experience as instructors, professors, program directors, and medical consultants. Participants received training mainly from individuals practicing psychiatry, theology, or medicine.

On the average, respondents reported providing seven formal consultations, nineteen informal consultations, and four interpretation-of-policy consultations a year. Data were gathered concerning the years 1980 to 1984. The busiest year for consultations of all types was 1983.

Although most of the respondents reported keeping records or case notes at least some of the time, a large majority said they chose not to keep records, on occasion, because of the possibility that the notes could be discovered by unauthorized persons, or brought into courtroom proceedings. More than half of the participants said they regularly wrote in patient charts; some did so only upon request. The majority exercised some jurisdiction in specific ethics issues, and hospital staffs are often obliged to follow that advice. Ethics consultants consulted most frequently with other ethicists.

The issues encountered most frequently by the ethics consultants were removal of life supports and refusal of resuscitation or treatment. Issues posing the most frequent difficulty for the respondents were full disclosure, organ donor issues, and genetic counseling. Most respondents served as resource persons for interpretation of institutional policy on an occasional-to-frequent basis.

Collaboration

Half of the participants reported having one or more collaborators. The most frequently used collaborators were administrators, internists, lawyers, and psychiatrists. Neonatologists, other ethicists, and clinical investigators were most often named as sources of referral, with the highest frequency of referrals coming from clinical investigators. Slightly over half of the 38 participants said they used a psychiatrist for consultation and 16 percent said they used a psychiatrist as a major collaborator. Fifty percent of the psychiatrists-as-collaborators came from departments of psychiatry, and the other 50 percent from liaison-consultation services. Their services were most frequently relied upon for examinations of competence.

Psychiatrists were used as consultants mostly on a rare-to-occasional basis; on the average about 15 times per year. Thirty-one percent of the participants saw a psychiatrist for emotional problems attendant to ethics consultation, most often concerning emotional problems of patients.

The specialties of other collaborators included medicine, theology, and law. Colleagues in philosophy were named least often as a source of collaboration. Contacts with collaborators from specialties other than psychiatry averaged once per month.

ADDITIONAL ANALYSES

Additional analyses, in the form of matrices, were conducted to suggest possible relationships among initial findings.

In comparing number of consultations, by respondent discipline, respondents in philosophy and ethics accounted for the highest number of total consultations, and respondents in law and education had the fewest consultations. Informal consultations were conducted far more often than were formal or interpretive consultations.

Philosophy was the discipline represented most often among the respondents and most of those in philosophy were employed by universities. However, the work setting accounting for the highest number of consultations was hospitals. Universities accounted for the fewest consultations.

Respondents were compared on frequency of difficulty with ethical issues, with respect to training and previous ethics consultation experience. The formal training of respondents had little association with the manner in which they perceived the frequency of difficulty with issues. Respondents with and without formal training ranked most issues, overall, as "occasionally difficult." Similar results were found when participants were compared on the basis of previous related experience. However, when respondents were compared in terms of the number of years in their current positions, a different picture was presented. The number of years spent in their current positions seemed to affect the frequency of difficulty perceived regarding issues in general. Respondents with the fewest years in service, 0 to 5 years, rated most issues as "never difficult" to "rarely difficult," while more seasoned veterans rated most issues as "occasionally difficult." The number of years the respondents had spent in the same position was also associated with the specific issues perceived as being most frequently difficult.

Respondents were also compared in terms of frequency of issue difficulty and the number of consultations they had performed. Regardless of the number of consultations they had performed, most respondents rated most issues as "occasionally difficult." However, the number of consultations did seem to be associated with specific issues regarded as having the most frequent difficulty.

Respondents were compared regarding source of collaboration and discipline. Respondents in philosophy had the greatest variety of collaborators. It was also found that respondents in different disciplines varied in their choice of collaborators.

Index

C

California, University of at Los
Angeles: Department of
Medicine, 29; Medical Center,
29, 30; School of Nursing, 30
California, University of at San
Francisco, 71, 110–11;
Division of Medical Ethics, 2
Callahan, Daniel, 24, 128;
bioethical methodology, 40
Caplan, Arthur, 24
Caplan, Gerald, 102, 104
Carlton, Wendy: clinical
discussion, 23; clinical
judgment, 21; clinical
problems, 22
Cases, 2–7
Cassell, Eric J.: clinical context,
26; clinical-ethical decision
making, 24; clinical meaning,
21
CC. *See* Magnuson (Warren G.)
Clinical Center
Center for Bioethics (Montreal),
10
Chicago, University of, 28
Childress, James, 129
Churchill, Larry R., clinical
medicine, 25
Clinical: definition, 20–23;
history of the word, 20
Clinical caregivers, moral
reflection, 38
Clinical-ethical decision making,
23–24
Clinical ethicists. *See* Medical
ethicists
Clinical ethics. *See* Medical
ethics
Clouser, K. Danner, 24; teaching
ethics, 27
Columbia University, College of
Physicians and Surgeons, 27

Consultants. *See* Ethics
consultants
Consultation: clinical, 100;
consultee-centered, 102–4;
liaison psychiatry, 105–6;
models, 102–6; nonmedical
disciplines, 105. *See also* Ethics
consultation
Consulting roles: action, 41;
advocacy, 42–43; analysis,
39–40; analysis assumptions,
50–51; answers, 39–40;
critique, 43–44; impartiality,
42–43; interpretation, 43–44;
reflection, 41

D

Declaration of Helsinki, 67
Department of Health and
Human Services (DHHS), 69,
121; legal rules and norms,
157
Department of Health,
Education, and Welfare
(DHEW), 68–69
DHEW. *See* Department of
Health, Education, and
Welfare
DHHS. *See* Department of
Health and Human Services
DNR. *See* Do-not-resuscitate
Do-not-resuscitate (DNR) orders,
141–42, 145
Dyck, Arthur J., medical ethics,
28

E

Eberhard Foundation, 2
Engelhardt, H. Tristram, Jr.,
128
Ethical issues in medicine,
newsletter, 30
Ethical problems: physicians' part

T–W

About the Editors

JOHN C. FLETCHER, PH.D. is Director of the Center for Biomedical Ethics at the Health Sciences Center, University of Virginia. Along with Albert R. Jonsen, he convened the First National Conference on Ethics Consultation in Health Care in 1985. He directs a 12-member Ethics Consultation Service at the University of Virginia's Hospital. From 1977 until 1987, he served as Chief of the Bioethics Program at the Warren G. Magnuson Clinical Center, National Institutes of Health, Bethesda, Maryland.

NORMAN QUIST has written and edited several publications on bioethics. He is President of University Publishing Group, in Frederick, Maryland, where he has developed books and journals in bioethics, health policy, and law.

ALBERT R. JONSEN, PH.D. is Professor of Ethics in Medicine and Chairman of the Department of Medical History and Ethics, School of Medicine, University of Washington. He is coauthor, with Mark Siegler and William Winslade, of *Clinical Ethics*. He was a member of the President's Commission for the Study of Ethical Problems in Medicine.